# Biochemical & Medicinal Chemistry Series

*Series Editor*
**JOHN MANN**
*Department of Chemistry, University of Reading*

*Titles in this series*

Neuropharmacology
T. W. STONE

An Introduction to Biotransformations in Organic Chemistry
JAMES R. HANSON

Bacteria and Antibacterial Agents
JOHN MANN AND M. JAMES C. CRABBE

Biochemical & Medicinal Chemistry Series

# Neuropharmacology

**T. W. STONE**

*Pharmacology Laboratories*
*Division of Neuroscience and Biomedical Systems*
*University of Glasgow*

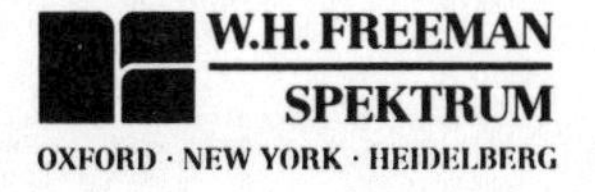

W.H. FREEMAN
SPEKTRUM
OXFORD · NEW YORK · HEIDELBERG

W. H. Freeman and Company Limited
20 Beaumont Street, Oxford OX1 2NQ
41 Madison Avenue, New York, NY 10010

British Library Cataloguing in Publication Data
A catalogue record for this book is available from the British Library.

Library of Congress Cataloging-in-Publication Data
Stone, T. W.
Neuropharmacology / T. W. Stone.
p. cm. — (biochemical and medicinal chemistry series)
Includes bibliographical references and index.
ISBN 0-7167-4510-0
1. Neuropharmacology. 2. Neurotransmitters. 3. Neurotransmitter receptors
I. Title II. Series.
[DNLM: 1. Central Nervous System Agents—pharmacology.
2. Central Nervous System Diseases—drug therapy. QV 76.5 S881n 1995]
RM315.S8925 1995 615'.78—dc20 DNLM/DLC for Library of Congress 95-4264 CIP



Set by Keyword Publishing Services
Printed by Bell & Bain Limited

# Contents

# Preface

This book is an introductory text on neuropharmacology. It may be viewed as an introduction or background reading for undergraduate or postgraduate students taking pharmacology as a component of their science (pharmacology, physiology, biochemistry, molecular biology, neuroscience) or medical degree, or needing elements of neuropharmacology for a Masters or Doctoral programme. It may be useful as the basis of a lecture or tutorial series, allowing a teacher to develop some topics in depth while permitting the student to become acquainted with most areas of neuropharmacology in their private reading. The book may also find use as a revision aid and refresher text.

The book has been written within the major constraint of length imposed on the volumes in this series. This has been a difficult and frustrating task, omitting much detail I would like to have included, and adopting a very concise and simplistic style of presentation. Nevertheless, I hope that most students will find this conciseness a help rather than a hindrance, and for the more interested students it will initiate that process of self-education and exploration in other sources, which is the aim of all teachers. Even with this constraint, most chapters have been written to be largely self-contained, or with specific cross-references. This results in elements of repetition, though these will greatly assist contextual retention of important points if the whole volume is read.

Pharmacology is essentially a biological subject, and the emphasis here is on human pharmacology, but a knowledge of molecular structures is essential to fully appreciate and understand the niceties of drug–receptor interactions. Examples of molecular structures are therefore included throughout, with several more detailed sections on structure–activity relationships.

Finally, I am immensely grateful to colleagues who read early drafts of chapters: Drs F. C. Boyle, M. J. Brodie, M. J. Higgins, D. G. MacGregor, T. C. Muir, D. Pollock and W. S. Wilson, to Ian Ramsden and Jane Grant for their patience and care in medical illustration, and my wife Anne for her continual encouragement.

# Abbreviations

|  |  |
|---|---|
| **A/E** | Adrenaline/epinephrine |
| **ACh** | Acetylcholine |
| **AChE** | Acetylcholinesterase |
| **AMPA** | α-Amino-3-hydroxy-5-methyl-4-isoxazolopropionic acid |
| **AT** | Angiotensin |
| **ATP** | Adenosine triphosphate |
| **BBB** | Blood–brain barrier |
| **BZ** | Benzodiazepine |
| **CCK** | Cholecystokinin |
| **CN** | Cranial nerves |
| **CNS** | Central nervous system |
| **COMT** | Catechol-*O*-methyltransferase |
| **CSF** | Cerebrospinal fluid |
| **Cyclic AMP** | Adenosine cyclic-3′5′-monophosphate |
| **Cyclic GMP** | Guanosine cyclic-3′5′-monophosphate |
| **DAG** | Diacylglycerol |
| **DOPA** | 3,4-dihydroxyphenylalanine |
| $E_{Na}$ | Equilibrium potential for sodium |
| **EJP** | Excitatory junction potential |
| **EPP** | End-plate potential |
| **EPS** | Extrapyramidal (Parkinsonian) symptoms |
| **EPSP** | Excitatory postsynaptic potential |
| $gCa^{++}$ | Calcium conductance (or permeability) |
| $gK^{+}$ | Potassium conductance (or permeability) |
| $gNa^{+}$ | Sodium conductance (or permeability) |
| $G_i$, $G_o$, $G_q$ | G-proteins |
| **GABA** | Gamma-aminobutyric acid |
| **GAD** | Glutamate decarboxylase |
| **GDP** | Guanosine diphosphate |
| **GTP** | Guanosine triphosphate |
| **I** | Current |
| $I_M$ | 'M' current |
| **IJP** | Inhibitory junction potential |
| **IP3** | Inositol triphosphate |
| **IPSP** | Inhibitory postsynaptic potential |
| **ISO** | Isoprenaline (isoproterenol; isopropyl-NA/NE) |
| **LC** | Locus coeruleus |
| **LSD** | Lysergic acid diethylamide |
| **5HT** | 5-Hydroxytryptamine |
| **MAC** | Minimal alveolar concentration |
| **MAO** | Monoamine oxidase |
| **MDMA** | Methylene-dioxymethamphetamine ('ecstasy') |
| **MPTP** | 1-Methyl-4-phenyl-1,2,3,6-tetrahydropyridine |
| **mRNA** | messenger RNA |
| **NA/NE** | Noradrenaline/norepinephrine |
| **NANC** | Non-adrenergic, non-cholinergic |
| **NB** | Nucleus basalis |
| **NGF** | Nerve growth factor |
| **NMDA** | *N*-Methyl-D-aspartate |
| **NMJ** | Neuromuscular junction |
| **NO** | Nitric oxide |
| **NSAIDs** | Non-steroidal anti-inflammatory drugs |
| **PAG** | Periaqueductal grey matter |
| **PCP** | Phencyclidine ('angel dust') |
| **PIP2** | Phosphatidylinositol bisphosphate |
| **PKC** | Protein kinase C |
| **PLA2** | Phospholipase A2 |
| **PLC** | Phospholipase C |
| **REM** | Rapid eye movement sleep |
| **RN** | Raphe nuclei |
| **RNA** | Ribonucleic acid |
| **SRIF** | Somatotropin release inhibitory factor |
| **SST** | Somatostatin |
| **TAD** | Tricyclic antidepressants |
| **TRH** | Thyrotrophin releasing hormone |
| **VIP** | Vasoactive intestinal peptide |

Abbreviations appearing only in tables or figures are defined in the legends.

# 1 Neuronal communication: synaptic transmission

## Introduction

The nervous system of humans includes around 10 million million ($10^{13}$) nerve cells or **neurons** in the central nervous system (CNS, the brain and spinal cord). The CNS communicates with skeletal and visceral structures via peripheral nerves. The junctions between neurons in the CNS are known as **synapses** and between nerves and muscle or endocrine tissues as **neuroeffector junctions**. At most of these junctions communication is achieved by the liberation of a chemical substance—a **neurotransmitter**—which brings about highly specific changes in the following, postsynaptic, cell. Many drugs acting on the nervous system do so by interfering in some way with this process of synaptic transmission, and this chapter will therefore examine this process in some detail.

## The synapse

Some basic generalized features of neurons in the CNS are illustrated in Figure 1.1. Each nerve cell gives rise to a branching axon which may be only a few micrometres long, or around a metre long in the case of neurons in the cerebral cortex projecting to the lower spinal cord. It is the expanded terminals of these axonal branches which form the synapses. In the CNS the synaptic connections can be made anywhere upon the surface of the postsynaptic neuron, but most occur either on the cell body (soma) or on an expanded network of receiving fibres—the **dendrites**—extending from the soma. Each nerve cell in the brain and spinal cord may produce and be contacted by many hundreds of synapses.

Signalling from one neuron to another is achieved by means of an **action potential**. Nerve cells usually have a potential difference across their resting membrane of around 70 millivolts, the inside of the cell being negative with respect to the outside (Figure 1.2). This potential originates from the fact that sodium ions exist mainly outside the cell, and potassium ions mainly inside, but permeability to the latter is about ten times greater than to sodium. A small depletion of intracellular cations results which, together with the electrical capacitance of the membrane itself, results in the observed potential difference. A small increase in sodium permeability or decrease of potassium permeability will lead to a fall of membrane potential known as a **depolarization**

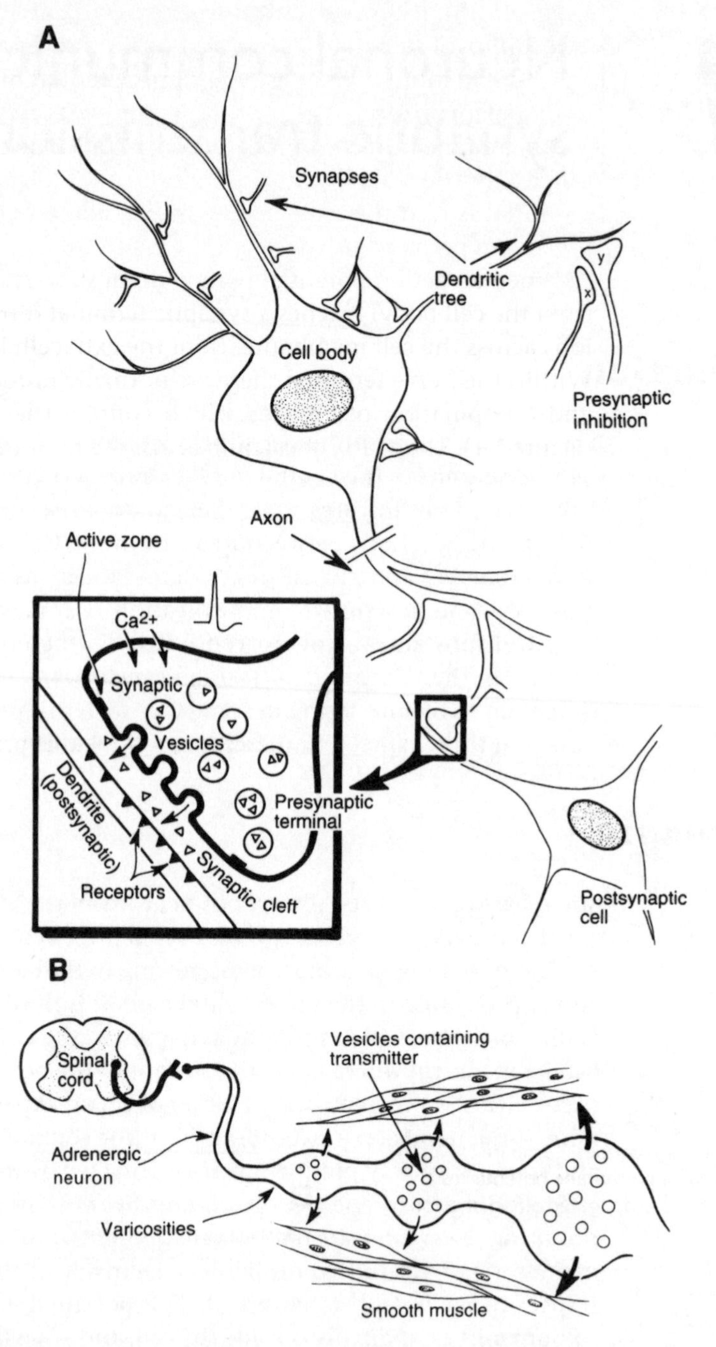


**Fig. 1.1**(A) A schematic representation of neurons and synapses in the central nervous system (CNS). Synapses can be made onto the cell body (soma) or dendrites of a neuron or onto other synaptic terminals (X onto Y). At a synapse, action potentials induce calcium influx which causes vesicles containing neurotransmitter to fuse with active zones, releasing their contents into the synaptic cleft by exocytosis. (B) In the peripheral nervous system and some CNS amino containing neurons, intercellular transmission occurs from varicosities which release transmitters into a relatively large extracellular space.

(Figure 1.2B). If depolarization reaches a critical 'threshold value', a relatively large influx of sodium occurs which causes a reversal of membrane potential to around +30 millivolts the equilibrium potential for sodium. (The **equilibrium potential** for an ion is the potential which exists across the cell membrane when the membrane is freely permeable to the ion.) The transient drop of membrane potential ('the spike') is the action potential (Figure 1.2C and D). Membrane potential is restored by a closure of the sodium channels and an increase of potassium permeability (Figure 1.2D).

When an action potential (which in most cases travels along the axon away from the cell body) reaches a synaptic terminal it triggers the influx of calcium ions across the cell membrane, from the extracellular fluid into the cytoplasm. Within the nerve terminal there are normally mitochondria, to supply energy, and a population of **vesicles** which contain the chemical neurotransmitter (Figure 1.1). The influx of calcium across the terminal membrane causes some of those vesicles to migrate towards 'active zones' located on portions of the

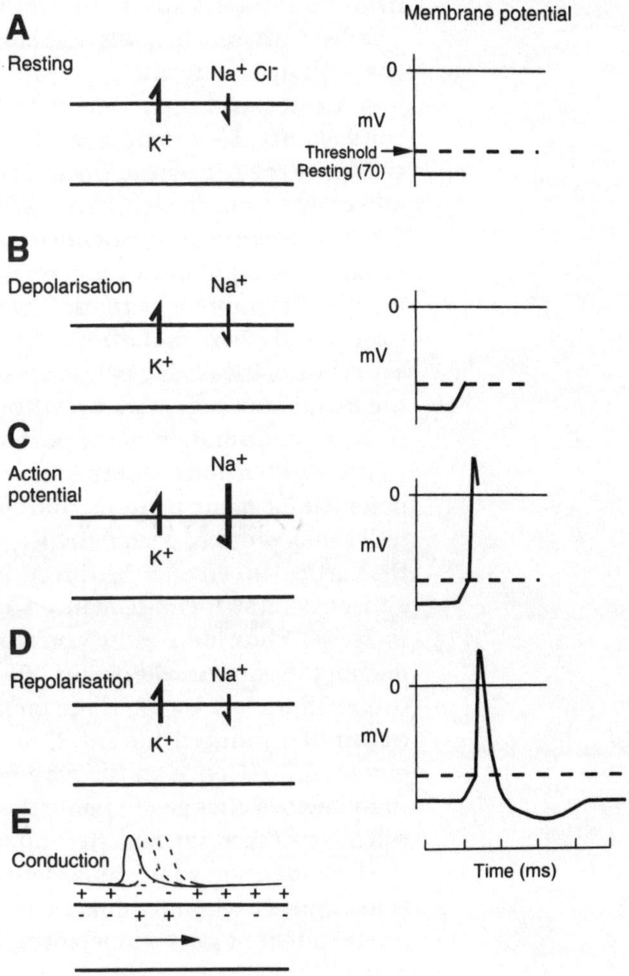

**Fig. 1.2** The effects of changing ionic permeability on membrane potential. (A) Increasing sodium permeability moves membrane potential towards the equilibrium potential for sodium ($E_{Na^+}$), producing a depolarization. (B) An increase of potassium permeability causes an efflux of potassium and moves membrane potential towards $E_{K^+}$, causing hyperpolarization. (C) Changes of chloride permeability have little effect on membrane potential, but by increasing overall membrane conductance, cause a reduced response to other ionic permeability changes (compare D with A). (E) The reversal of membrane potential as an action potential is propagated along an axon.

presynaptic membrane, where they fuse with the membrane and release their transmitter contents into the synaptic gap or cleft between the presynaptic and postsynaptic cells, a process known as **exocytosis**. The influx of calcium can be blocked by competing cations such as magnesium or cadmium. Because release is in the form of discrete 'packets' of transmitter from individual vesicles it is sometimes known as **quantal release**. Each vesicle or quantum may contain several thousand molecules of transmitter and several hundred quanta are often released by a single action potential. Even in the absence of calcium single vesicles occasionally collide with an active zone and release a single quantum of transmitter. The postsynaptic responses to these calcium-independent events are known as **miniature postsynaptic potentials** and are about 0.1 millivolt in size.

## What do neurotransmitters do?

Once released, the transmitter is able to act upon specialized receiving molecules, receptors, on the postsynaptic cell. The most obvious effects of neurotransmitters are to interact with receptor molecules which are directly coupled with ion channels, although some receptors can themselves form ionic channels upon activation.

A neurotransmitter which induces an increase of sodium or calcium conductance, for example, will induce an inward current in the postsynaptic cell (since the concentration and electrical gradients for these ions favour their movement from the extracellular space into the neuronal cytoplasm) (Figure 1.3A). This will cause a **depolarization** as the membrane potential is moved towards the equilibrium potential (e.g. $E_{Na}$). Conversely a transmitter which increased membrane permeability for potassium ions would cause an outward current and a **hyperpolarization** (Figure 1.3B). Some transmitters actually cause a decrease of the resting potassium channel conductance, an effect which moves the membrane potential away from $E_K$ and towards $E_{Na}$, i.e. a depolarization since the contribution of the potassium current is reduced.

The equilibrium potential for chloride ions is generally close to the resting potential for many neurons, and transmitters increasing chloride conductance ($gCl^-$) may produce a small hyperpolarization or depolarization depending on the particular cell and the direction of the chloride gradient (Figure 1.3C). In either case, however, the reduced total membrane resistance resulting from the increased chloride conductance, means that any superimposed change of membrane current will be less effective in changing the membrane potential (from Ohm's law $V = IR$; if the membrane resistance R is reduced then a given transmitter-induced current, I, must result in a smaller change of membrane potential, V). Hence, in the presence of an increased chloride conductance, a simultaneous change of membrane permeability to sodium (as in Figure 1.3A) will have a much smaller effect on membrane potential (Figure 1.3D).

These ideas are vitally important for understanding how the nervous system works. Since each individual neuron is contacted by many synapses acting on several different ion conductances, the membrane potential of each cell will be

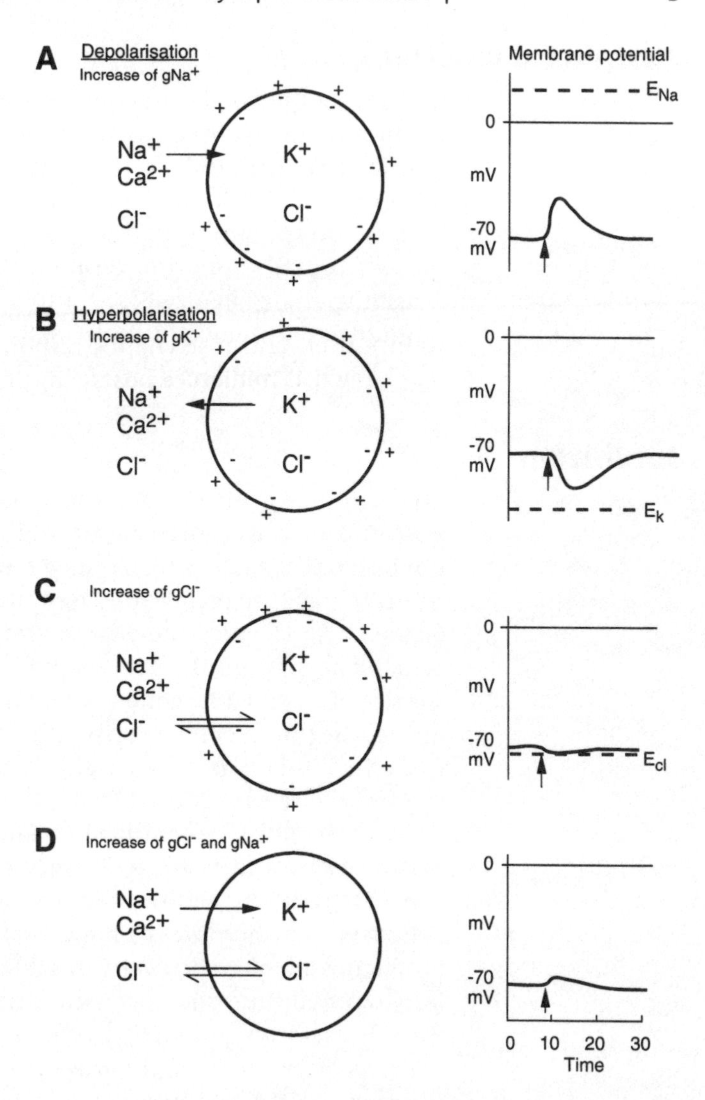


**Fig. 1.3** The membrane potential of neurons is determined by the differences of ionic concentration across the membrane, with higher sodium levels outside, and higher potassium inside, and the fact that the membrane is about ten-fold more permeable to potassium. Potassium can therefore move out of the cell faster than sodium can enter, generating a resting potential of around −70 mV (inside negative). (A) An agent which increases sodium conductance will tend to reduce these differences and cause depolarization (B) An agent which increases potassium conductance will increase the membrane potential towards the potassium equilibrium potential $E_K$. (C) A compound which increases chloride permeability may have little obvious effect on potential since $E_{cl}$ is near the resting potential. The decreased membrane resistance will still tend to short-circuit the effects of other agents, so that the effect seen in A would be greatly diminished, (D).

very unstable, fluctuating constantly in time as its membrane potential is altered by transmitters. Only when the membrane potential reaches a critical **threshold** value does the cell produce an **action potential** which can proceed to affect other cells in the nervous system. It is for this reason that transmitters producing depolarization are usually referred to as **excitatory**, and those producing hyperpolarization as **inhibitory**. The changes of membrane potential are correspondingly referred to as excitatory (e.g. Figure 1.3A) or inhibitory (e.g. Figure 1.3B) **postsynaptic potentials** (EPSPs or IPSPs). Transmitters which stabilize the membrane potential (as by increasing $gCl^-$), thus making it less excitable also function as inhibitory transmitters by diminishing the responses to other transmitters.

### Peripheral junctions

In the peripheral autonomic nervous system the changes of membrane potential induced by transmitters are referred to as excitatory or inhibitory **junction potentials** (EJPs or IJPs) since the relationship between presynaptic and postsynaptic membranes is often not as clearly defined as in the CNS. The transmitters containing portions of autonomic nerves take the form of swellings or 'varicosities' along the terminal length of the axons (Figure 1.1B). The transmitters are then released into a relatively large extracellular space, the postjunctional membrane being up to 1 micrometre away from the varicosity in some blood vessels and other smooth muscles.

### Inhibition

The inhibitory effects described so far are all mediated directly upon postsynaptic cells (**postsynaptic inhibition**) but there is an additional type of inhibition in the CNS which is mediated presynaptically. A synapse is formed by one cell upon the presynaptic terminal of another (see upper right portion of Figure 1.1A). The presynaptic inhibitory terminal X releases a transmitter which actually depolarizes the subsynaptic terminal Y. The effect of this is to reduce the size of an invading action potential, (which is only all-or-nothing as long as membrane properties are constant!) This reduces calcium influx into the terminal, since this is proportional to action potential size, and thus depresses transmitter release from terminal Y. The inhibition here is thus one of transmitter release rather than of neuronal excitability.

Already we can begin to understand how some disorders of the nervous system may arise and how they can be treated. Epilepsy, for example, includes disorders in which areas of the brain periodically become hyperexcitable, producing uncontrolled activity which can spread throughout the brain and lead to convulsions and unconsciousness. Part of the reason for this may be that there is excessive production of neurotransmitters causing depolarization of neurons. Treatment might then involve either preventing the transmitter interacting with receptors, by using an antagonistic drug, or administering agents which have the opposite, inhibitory, effect, reducing excitability by hyperpolarizing cells or increasing chloride conductance.

## Neurotransmitters

Each neurotransmitter must have processes for its synthesis, storage, release and removal after release, and drugs can act on the nervous system by interfering with any of these processes. In addition most neurotransmitters interact with several different receptors, providing an opportunity for the design of drugs which act selectively on only one type. This clearly brings the advantage of introducing fewer effects on other receptors which may be involved in unwanted side effects of the drugs.

## Criteria for transmitter identification

Detailed consideration of individual neurotransmitters will be left for later chapters. First, though, it is important to realize that because the nervous system is so complex and transmitters are localized to such a limited compartment as synaptic vesicles, it is extraordinarily difficult to determine which of the thousands of substances present in the nervous system is indeed a transmitter. The following criteria have become generally accepted as indicating that a substance may be a neurotransmitter. For some compounds only two or three criteria have been satisfied.

### Presence of a neurotransmitter

It may seem obvious that a neurotransmitter should be present in the nervous system, but this simplest of criteria hides a multitude of problems. Many substances, for example, may fulfil several roles in cells. Amino acids such as glutamate are often important intermediates on vital biochemical pathways and are, of course, used in the synthesis of peptides and proteins. Conversely cellular catabolism will release substantial quantities of glutamate. It is not sufficient, therefore, to show that a candidate transmitter is present, but it should be localized to nerve terminals, and ideally should be shown to be present in synaptic vesicles. The former can be achieved easily because when nervous tissue is homogenized under certain well-defined conditions the synaptic terminals break off from their axons and seal themselves into almost spherical entities known as 'synaptosomes'. These can then be studied directly or disrupted by chemicals or hypertonic solutions to release their vesicular contents for analysis.

With more refined separation methods the synaptic vesicle fraction can be retained intact for analysis. Even here, though, difficulties may be encountered. It proved exceedingly difficult to prepare synaptic vesicles which contained the amino acid transmitters such as glutamate. Although this has now been achieved, evidence for the presence of glutamate in vesicles was based on the demonstration of an avid uptake system for glutamate into vesicles.

An alternative method of demonstrating the presence of a transmitter is to use an antibody to it or its synthesizing enzyme, which can be linked to a stain or radioactive marker. Such techniques of histochemistry and immunocytochemistry can then be used to visualize the molecules of interest in thin sections of the nervous system.

A further problem with the criterion of presence is that some transmitters may not be present in their released, active form. Several peptides, for example, are synthesized and stored as large precursor molecules and are only formed enzymatically at the time of release, or indeed after release of the precursor. This criterion, therefore, has to be considered in parallel with the following points.

### Synthesis of neurotransmitters

Most neurotransmitters are synthesized by the neurons which release them and the demonstration of appropriate enzymes either by biochemical or immunohistochemical techniques has proved to be a valuable way of identifying neurons releasing a particular transmitter. In the case of some peptides, as mentioned above, the ability to produce the peptide at an appropriate time and place may actually be a more valid criterion than the presence of peptide itself. It must also be realized that some transmitters are not synthesized specifically for transmission. Again, using the example of glutamate, this amino acid is both synthesized and catabolized in metabolic pathways quite unrelated to neurotransmission.

## Release of neurotransmitters

A neurotransmitter must by definition be released from neurons. This can often be demonstrated by taking sections of brain or peripheral tissue, or preparing synaptosomes, and showing that depolarization by high concentrations of extracellular potassium, electrical stimulation or the plant alkaloid veratridine (from the Veratrum, or periwinkle, plant) will cause the efflux of the suspected transmitter. Since synaptic transmission *in situ* normally appears to be dependent on calcium influx into the presynaptic terminal, it is essential that at least a proportion of the transmitter candidate is also released in a calcium dependent manner. As noted above it is important also to consider that the released material may be a precursor form of the transmitter. It may be possible to study release of the natural transmitter molecule or of a radioactive form of it which behaves identically in the neurons.

Release may also be examined *in vivo* using microdialysis in which a fine probe, consisting of two concentric tubes about 100 micrometres in diameter, is inserted into a region of the nervous system. A physiological solution (containing $Na^+$, $Cl^-$, $K^+$, $Ca^{2+}$ and $Mg^{2+}$ can then be pumped along one tube to the tip of the probe where it will mix with a minute volume of extracellular fluid and then be sucked out along the second tube for analysis. The tip of the probe is covered by a dialysis membrane so that small molecules such as transmitters can pass into the probe from where they are pumped out for analysis.

## Removal of neurotransmitters

If the nervous system is to function with speed and precision it is essential that neurotransmitters have a relatively transient effect, being removed in order for another neurotransmitter signal to be processed within milliseconds. Transmitters may be removed in several ways. Probably the most rapid is enzyme destruction as in the case of acetylcholine (ACh) which can be hydrolysed by **acetylcholinesterase** (AChE), closely associated with the receptor molecules in some postsynaptic membranes. This enzyme can destroy about 10,000 molecules of ACh every second. Another method of removal is for cells around the synaptic cleft (including presynaptic terminals, postsynaptic cells and supporting cells such as glia) to transport the transmitter rapidly across their cell membranes into the cytoplasm where it can be safely repackaged into vesicles or destroyed over a period of time. Such uptake is normally by active transport (energy-dependent) and is dependent on external sodium concentrations.

### Pharmacology of neurotransmitters

One of the most important criteria for a putative neurotransmitter to fulfil is that of identity of action. In other words, the effects produced by the candidate compound should mimic the effects of the natural transmitter released from the synaptic terminals. Equally, both should show the same pharmacology, being potentiated by inhibitors of uptake or metabolism, or blocked by the same antagonists. Techniques such as microiontophoresis allow substances to be applied from micropipettes, with tips only 1or 2 micrometres, in size, to individual cells, thus helping to exclude effects of the compounds on distant sites or cells. It may still be difficult to meet this criterion fully, however, if a synapse releases transmitter onto part of the dendritic tree. This may produce changes of membrane properties which cannot readily be studied with intracellular electrodes in or near the cell body.

An extension of this criterion is that of denervation supersensitivity. Loss of receptor activation, either due to neuronal damage or the chronic presence of antagonists, often results in an increase in the number (up-regulation) of the receptors so that responses to agonists are increased relative to control cells. This change should be observed both for the endogenous neurotransmitter and for the experimentally applied exogenous candidate compound.

## Receptor structure

Every neurotransmitter produces its effects by interacting with a **receptor** molecule in the cell membrane but until relatively recently little was known of the precise structure of receptor molecules or how they induce changes in the postjunctional cell.

If a ligand can be identified with a very high affinity for a particular receptor, then that ligand can be chemically bound to the stationary phase of a chromatography column. When a homogenate of appropriate cells is now passed over the column, some of the receptor will bind to the ligand and can thus be separated from other cellular components. The sequence of amino acids in the purified receptor can then be determined. The complete structure of one receptor, the beta-2-adrenoceptor for catecholamines (Chapter 3) is illustrated in Figure 1.4).

In practice most molecular pharmacologists now obtain pure receptor preparations by an extension of this technique. Once part of the receptor structure has been obtained, it is possible to predict the nucleotide sequence of the messenger RNA (mRNA) and DNA which could have coded for that protein. An oligonucleotide probe with about 25 bases can then be synthesized to bind with the naturally occurring nucleic acid. Using a preparation of cells in which the DNA has been enzymically split into pieces (a cDNA library) the synthetic oligonucleotide can be used to identify portions of the DNA corresponding to the receptor protein. Those DNA fragments can then be reproduced by using the polymerase chain reaction in which a polymerase enzyme and others are used to copy the DNA sequence several million times. The resulting DNA or mRNA is then injected into cells such as the oocytes of the *Xenopus* toad. These cells treat

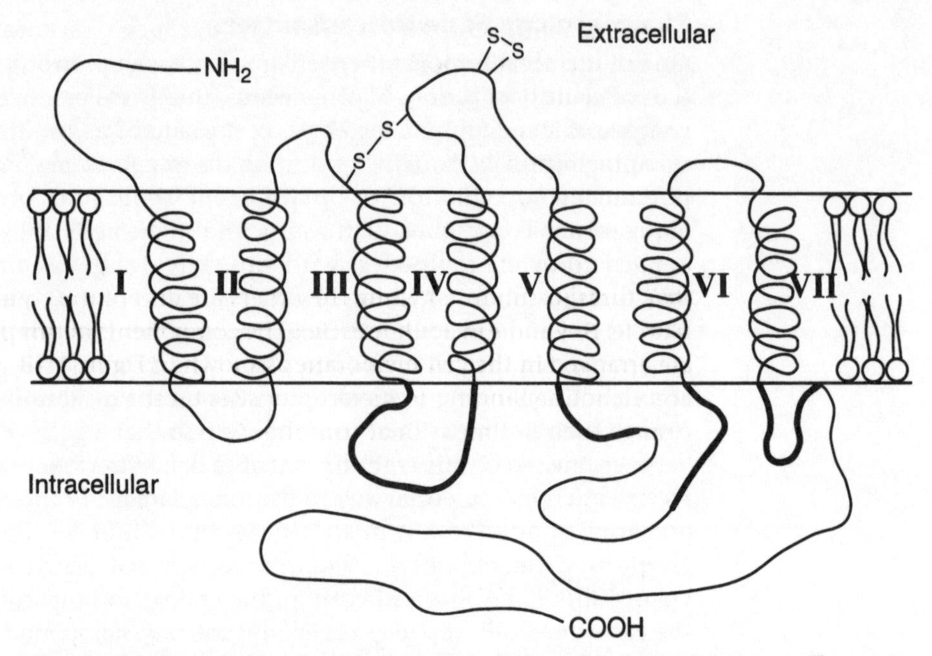


**Fig. 1.4** A schematic diagram showing the outline structure of the beta-adrenoceptor. The receptor has seven trans-membrane spanning regions (I–VII) with an amino terminus portion in the extracellular space and a C-terminal portion in the cytosol. The thicker-marked segments of the intracellular loops indicate regions known to be involved in the interactions with G-proteins.

the foreign nucleic acid as their own and transcribe it into receptor protein. Once the receptors are inserted into the cell membrane their properties can be studied in detail.

Using this technique it has been discovered that what were once considered to be single receptors actually exist in several different subtypes. Information on these will be presented where appropriate throughout this book.

Much of the detailed knowledge we now have about receptors (e.g. Figure 1.4) comes from experiments in which a modified probe was used to initiate synthesis of a receptor population. This can introduce an error into the receptor sequence and study of the effect this has on receptor function can provide much information on ligand binding sites or receptor coupling to other cellular systems. The introduction of such errors is known as **site-directed mutagenesis**.

## Receptor superfamilies

It has become clear that all the receptors studied until now fall into four groups or **superfamilies**. Within each group there is substantial sequence homology (similarity of amino acid sequence) suggesting a common evolutionary origin.

### Ligand-gated channels

Some receptors are organized so that when activated they directly open an ionic channel. As an example, the nicotinic receptors for acetylcholine (Chapter 2) consist of five separate molecules or **subunits**. Each of these subunits consists of a protein, about 500 amino acids in length, which crosses back and forth across the cell membrane so that there are four transmembrane spanning segments of the molecule (Figure 1.5). (The molecule actually crosses five times, but only the hydrophobic regions, labelled I–IV are considered as true, integral membrane-spanning regions.) The fifth intramembrane segment has one face of its $\alpha$-helix structure hydrophobic and one face hydrophilic. The latter face forms the lining of the (aqueous) ion channel through the cell membrane.

Each complete receptor is made up of five subunits. Two have identical structures ($\alpha$-subunits) while the others are different ($\beta$, $\gamma$ and $\delta$ in embryonic muscle; $\beta$, $\gamma$ and $\varepsilon$ in adult muscle). The components of this pentameric receptor are arranged in the cell membrane as shown in Figure 1.5B. When activated by acetylcholine binding to its receptor sites on the $\alpha$-subunits, the five subunits change their 3-dimensional conformation so that a pore or channel is created between them. It is through this channel that small ions can pass (Chapter 2). As well as nicotinic receptors, receptors for the amino acids GABA, glycine and NMDA (Chapter 4) form ligand-gated channels.

### G-protein coupled receptors

The second superfamily of receptors are not coupled directly to ion channels, but to a family of intracellular proteins known as **G-proteins**. (This name comes from the fact that they are normally bound either to guanosine diphosphate (GDP) or triphosphate (GTP).)

The $\beta$2-receptor illustrated in Figure 1.4 is a good example of a G-protein coupled receptor. All members of this superfamily possess seven transmembrane spanning regions. Different members of one receptor group (e.g. $\beta$-receptors) show a high degree of homology between their membrane-spanning portions,

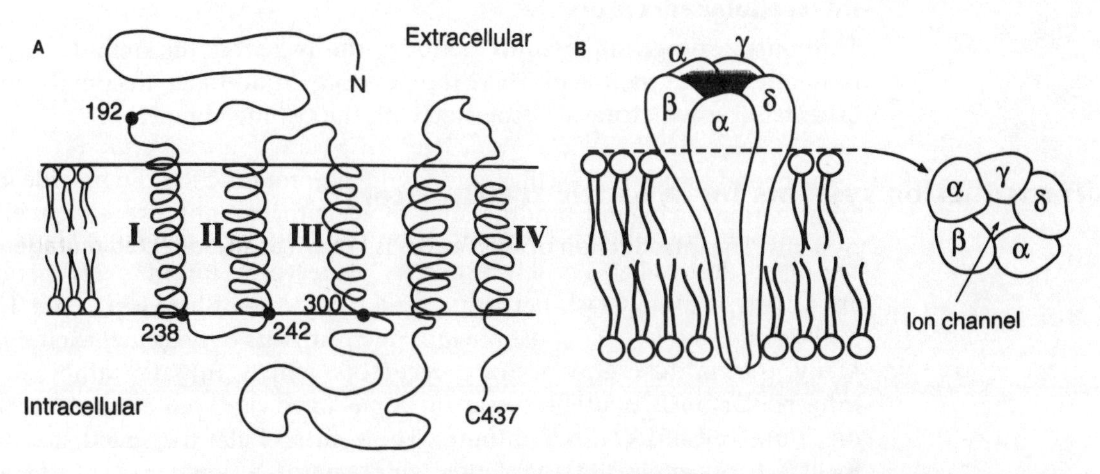


**Fig. 1.5** (A) A diagram of the nicotinic acetylcholine receptor, which contains 437 amino acids and consists of four main transmembrane segments (I–IV). (B) A three-dimensional impression of the receptor seen in longitudinal and transverse sections to illustrate the arrangement of the five subunits, and the creation of a pore or channel between them for the passage of cations when activated by acetylcholine.

with greater diversity in the structure of the extracellular and intracellular sections. This is presumably because the agonist binding site, one of the most critical parts of the receptor, lies within the membrane-spanning region.

When an agonist binds to the receptor, a conformation change occurs in the receptor as a result of which the intracellular loop interacts with a G-protein. This would normally be associated with GDP, but on interacting with the receptor, GDP is exchanged for GTP. In this form the G-protein can interact with other proteins and enzymes (or **transduction systems**) within the cell as described below. Other members of the G-protein coupled superfamily include receptors for dopamine and 5-hydroxytryptamine, and the muscarinic receptors for acetylcholine.

### G-proteins

More than twenty types of G-protein are now recognized, though the effects of some have not yet been fully characterized. In general they can be classified into three groups. Members of the $G_i$ group are able to inhibit the enzyme adenylate cyclase, and some are coupled to ionic channels. The $G_s$ group activates adenylate cyclase and in the heart can open cation channels. The $G_q$ group is responsible for activating phospholipase C, opening some potassium channels and closing some calcium channels.

### Tyrosine kinase linked receptors

The third receptor superfamily includes those which contain or activate intracellular tyrosine kinases. This results in phosphorylation of the tyrosine groups in target proteins. These receptors respond primarily to agents having long-term effects on cell growth and development—the growth factors—and are beyond the scope of this book.

### Intracellular receptors

The fourth known superfamily includes the receptors for steroids, thyroid hormones and retinoic acid. These receptors are intracellular, in contrast to the other families which are all associated with the cell membrane.

## Transduction systems for synaptic transmitters

The transduction systems for synaptic transmitters are outlined in Figure 1.6. The direct electrical effects of transmitters, via receptors linked to ion channels, are usually relatively fast, occurring on a time scale of between 1 and 1,000 milliseconds and are the most obvious determinants of neuronal excitability. Many transmitters also activate receptors which initiate rather slower intracellular biochemical processes, often mediated via G-proteins, which occur on a time scale of seconds or minutes. These intracellular **transduction systems** include, for example, the stimulation (via $G_s$) or inhibition (via $G_i$) of **adenylate cyclase**, an enzyme system which catalyses the conversion of ATP (adenosine triphosphate) into **cyclic AMP** (adenosine cyclic 3′, 5′-monophosphate) (Figure 1.6A), or the modulation of guanylate cyclase which performs a similar service for guanosine triphosphate (GTP) and **cyclic GMP**.

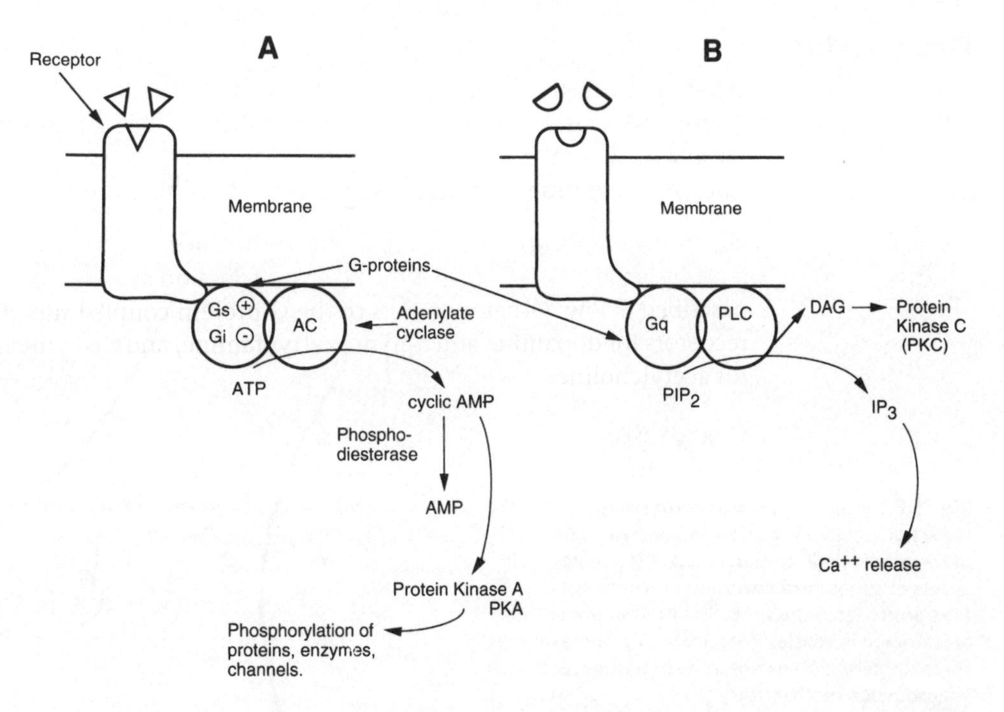


**Fig. 1.6** Second messenger signal transduction systems operated by neurotransmitter action. (A) The adenylate cyclase system leading to cyclic adenosine monophosphate (cyclic AMP) and activation of protein kinase A (PKA). (B) The phosphatidylinositol system leading to inositol trisphosphate (IP3) and calcium release, and diacylglycerol (DAG) and activation of protein kinase C (PKC).

Several transmitters can also activate **phospholipase C**, which catalyses the hydrolysis of phosphatidylinositol bisphosphate (PIP2) into **1,4,5-inositol trisphosphate** (IP3) and **diacylglycerol** (DAG) (Figure 1.6B). IP3 is able to release calcium from intracellular storage sites such as the endoplasmic reticulum, while DAG activates protein kinase C (PKC), an enzyme system responsible for phosphorylating other proteins, enzymes and ion channels within the cells or membranes. If the targets for PKC in a particular cell include ion channel proteins, then a change of ionic conductance may be produced by this route, though clearly with a rather slow time course.

It is important to emphasize at this point the importance of biochemical second messengers such as cyclic AMP or IP3. Firstly, they can be instrumental in initiating changes of cell growth or function by complex pathways involving calcium, nuclear transcription factors and genetic changes. This means that neurotransmitters and related agents (including drugs) may have long-term influences on the structure and function of the nervous system.

Secondly, these biochemical pathways provide an excellent means by which neurotransmitters can affect each other's activity by acting at the genetic level to change the number or type of receptors or ion channels. Such interactions are a major reason why the nervous system is such a complex and challenging organ to understand.

## Drug action

Already it will be apparent that drugs can potentially interfere with synaptic transmission in several ways, and many of these will be introduced in the course of this book. In the meantime, Figure 1.7 summarizes ten of the most common sites at which drugs can act at peripheral or central synapses.

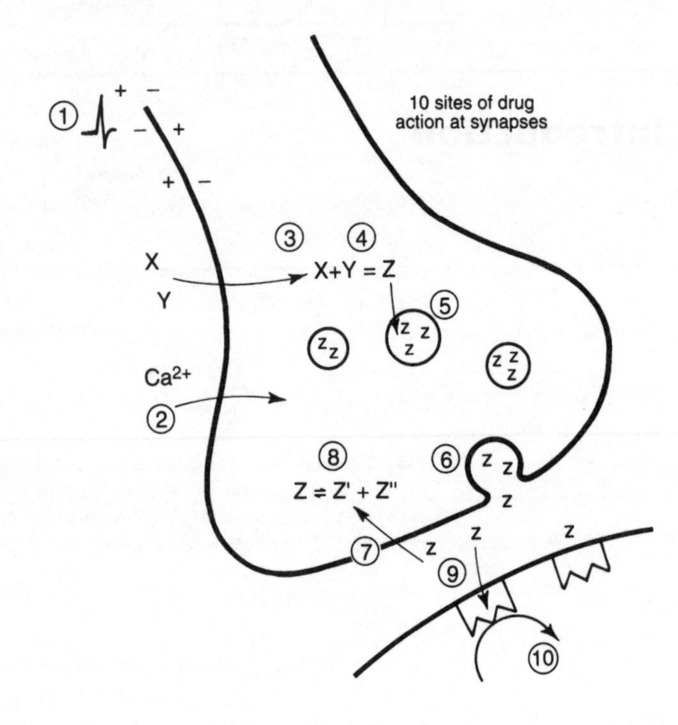


**Fig. 1.7** Ten sites of drug action at synapses: (1) action potential invasion and depolarization of the terminal; (2) calcium influx; (3) altered access or structure of transmitter precursors; (4) transmitter synthesis; (5) transmitter uptake and storage in vesicles; (6) release; (7) reuptake; (8) metabolism; (9) receptors; (10) postreceptor (transduction mechanisms).

# 2 Somatic nervous system: the neuromuscular junction

## Introduction

The term neuromuscular junction (nmj) is very specific. It refers to the synapses between motor nerves and skeletal (somatic, striated or 'voluntary') muscle. At these synapses, the neurons release a simple quaternary amine, **acetylcholine** (ACh) as their neurotransmitter. These nerves are referred to as **cholinergic**.

## Acetylcholine

Acetylcholine (ACh) (Figure 2.1) is synthesized within motor axon terminals, from choline and acetylcoenzyme A, by the enzyme choline acetyltransferase (Figure 2.2). After synthesis, ACh is stored in synaptic vesicles and released by exocytosis, as described in Chapter 1, following the influx of calcium across the nerve terminal membrane. After release, the ACh diffuses rapidly across the synaptic gap and acts upon its receptors. Closely associated with ACh receptors is the enzyme **acetylcholinesterase** (AChE) which inactivates ACh by hydrolysis, within 1 or 2 milliseconds, into choline ana acetate (Figure 2.2). The choline is then recycled—it is taken up back into the nerve terminal by a high affinity transport system and reused ACh synthesis.

### Acetylcholine receptors (nicotinic)

Acetylcholine can act on several different types of receptor in the body, but those located on skeletal muscle can also be activated by the tobacco alkaloid **nicotine** (Figure 2.1). The receptors are therefore referred to as **nicotinic** receptors and are normally concentrated in a specialized region of membrane known as the end-plate where there are around 10,000 per square micrometre. They spread outside the end-plate region if muscle is denervated.

Each receptor consists of five protein subuits, two $\alpha$, one $\beta$, one $\gamma$, one $\delta$, arranged in a rosette formation (Chapter 1; Figure 1.5) which span the thickness of the membrane. When ACh binds to its attachment sites on the two $\alpha$-subunits of the receptor, a conformation change is initiated which creates a channel, or pore, across the muscle membrane. This receptor-operated channel is rather unselective and most cations, including $Na^+$, $Ca^{2+}$ and $K^+$ can pass through. The result is that in response to ACh the membrane potential at the

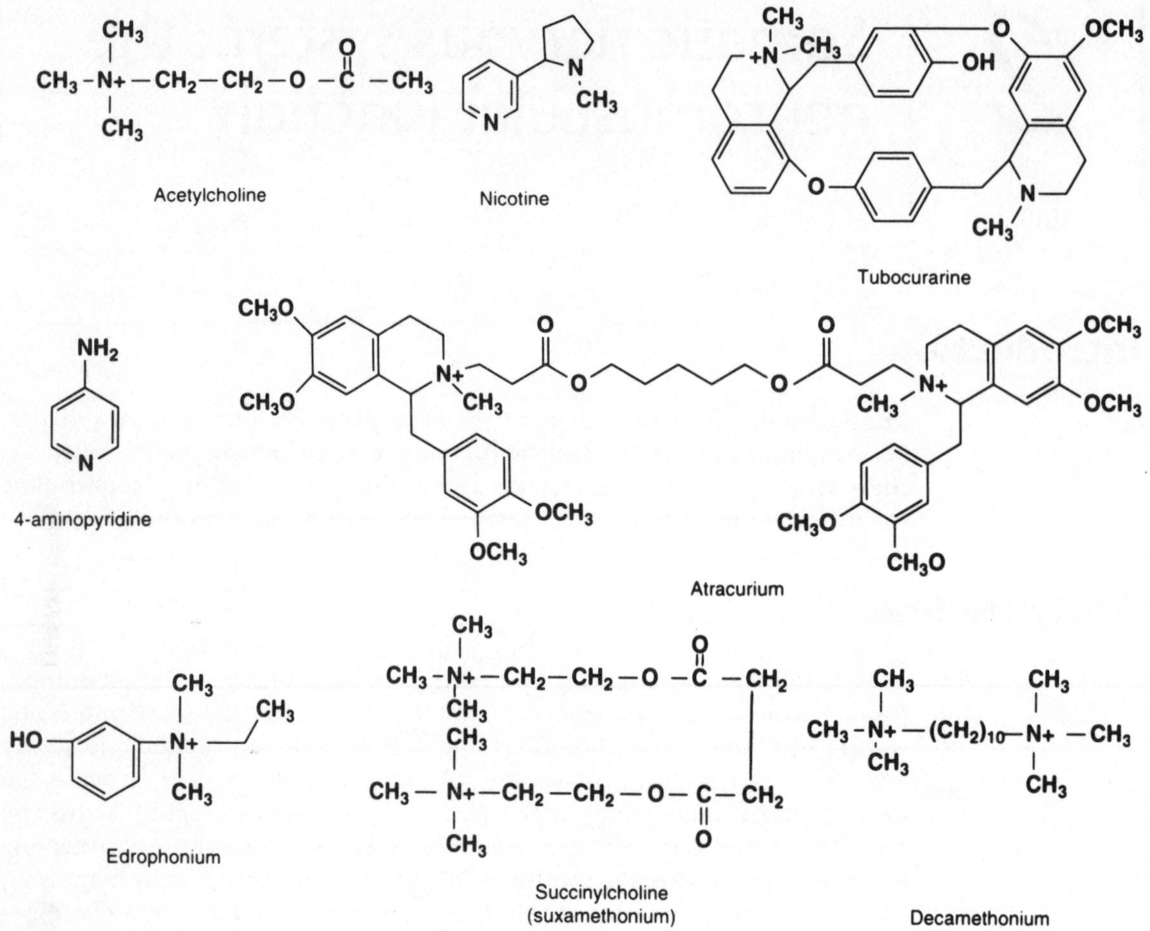

Acetylcholine

Nicotine

Tubocurarine

4-aminopyridine

Atracurium

Edrophonium

Succinylcholine (suxamethonium)

Decamethonium

**Fig. 2.1** Structural formulae of some cholinomimetic agents: acetylcholine, nicotine, the neuromuscular blocking drugs succinlycholine and decamethonium, and the anticholinesterases dyflos and eserine.

end-plate falls by up to 60 millivolts. This ACh-induced depolarization is referred to as an **end-plate potential** and is analogous to the EPSP described for neurons in Chapter 1. The fall of membrane potential at the end-plate in turn causes a depolarization of adjacent muscle membrane. If depolarization is adequate, it opens voltage-operated channels which are selective for sodium, initiating an action potential which propagates to the sarcoplasmic reticulum to release calcium and cause muscle contraction (Figure 2.2).

# Drugs acting at the neuromuscular junction

## Compounds affecting ACh synthesis

The hemicholinium series of compounds interact with the membrane transporter for choline, preventing the salvage of choline from the synaptic cleft. Since the supply of choline is a major limiting factor in the synthesis of ACh this can lead to a virtual cessation of ACh synthesis. The vesicular content

Gallamine

Ecothiopate

Pancuronium

Neostigmine

DFP, dyflos

Eserine (physostigmine)

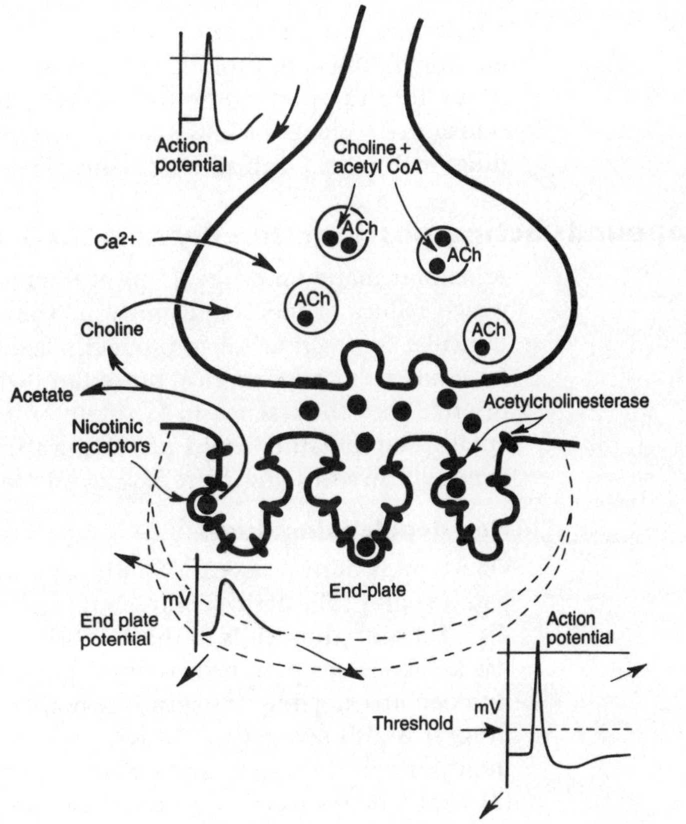


**Fig. 2.2** Summary of events at the skeletal neuromuscular junction. Following synthesis from choline and acetyl CoA, acetylcholine is released to act on postjunctional nicotinic receptors. Sufficient depolarization at the end-plate region initiates an action potential which causes muscle contraction. Acetylcholine is hydrolysed by acetylcholinesterase and choline is taken up into the terminals.

of ACh thus becomes severely depleted and synaptic transmission fails. Synthesis can also be inhibited by ACh analogues such as bromo-acetylcholine and triethylcholine, acting by a mechanism similar to the hemicholiniums.

## Compounds affecting ACh release

The release of ACh, like that of most transmitters, is dependent on calcium influx and can therefore be prevented by calcium removal or chelating agents, or by cations which block calcium channels (magnesium, cadmium, cobalt).

One of the bacteria causing food poisoning, *Clostridium botulinum*, manufactures a toxic molecule known as **botulinum toxin**. This blocks the release of ACh from axon terminals, probably by affecting calcium availability or effects, and causes widespread paralysis known as botulism. Conversely, the venom of the black widow spider disrupts the cholinergic synaptic vesicles causing a rapid, almost explosive, release of stored ACh, demonstrable as a storm of miniature end-plate potentials. The toxin also prevents storage of ACh in vesicles and, like botulinum toxin, causes widespread paralysis which can lead to death from respiratory failure. It may be necessary to place patients on life-support and artificial lung machines for several weeks until the toxins are eliminated and new vesicles synthesized.

A different group of substances able to facilitate neuromuscular transmission are the aminopyridines. **4-Aminopyridine**, for example, blocks potassium channels in nerve membranes. Since the efflux of $K^+$ contributes to repolarization and afterhyperpolarization in many cells, the effect of 4-aminopyridine is to prolong the action potential and thus increase calcium influx into the nerve terminals. This in turn results in a greater release of transmitter. Agents such as 4-aminopyridine have been explored as potential drugs in disorders such as myasthenia gravis and multiple sclerosis.

## Compounds acting postjunctionally and their clinical uses

A major demand for drugs acting at the neuromuscular junction is for agents which reduce or block transmission. The effect of this action is to decrease muscular contraction, i.e. to produce relaxation, something which is necessary for many medical or surgical procedures where, for example, a tube has to be inserted into the trachea to facilitate artificial respiration, or where surgery entails manipulating limbs or cutting through layers of muscle. The drugs which achieve this, muscle relaxants, are two main types.

### Non-depolarizing drugs

One type is derived from a South American arrow poison, curare, used to paralyse prey. The active compound is now available as **tubocurarine** (Figure 2.1). Tubocurarine binds to the ACh receptor and prevents the action of ACh itself. Tubocurarine has no agonist, depolarizing, effect itself; it is an example of non-depolarizing muscle relaxant or non-depolarizing neuromuscular blocking drug. It is also competitive, a term which, as in all fields of pharmacology, indicates that the block can be reversed by increasing the amount of agonist (ACh) around the receptor, since the agonist will then soon replace the blocking drug and restore transmission. Indeed if it is desirable to remove the block quickly after a surgical operation, or if an overdose of tubocurarine has been administered, the muscular paralysis can be reversed by using drugs which prevent the breakdown of ACh (see later) thus increasing its local concentration.

Other non-depolarizing neuromuscular blocking drugs in clinical use include **pancuronium** and **vecuronium** (the structures of which are based on the steroid nucleus; Figure 2.1), **gallamine** and **atracurium** (Figure 2.1). These are often preferred in clinical practice because tubocurarine has a number of actions which are often undesirable, including the ability to release histamine, causing bronchial and salivary secretions, and the danger of hypertension and bronchospasm in asthmatics. Tubocurarine is also able to block ganglionic synapses (see Chapter 3) resulting in hypotension and reduced gastrointestinal tone and motility. Pancuronium does not block ganglia or release histamine but it and gallamine can block ACh release and inhibitory muscarinic receptors in the heart, causing tachycardia (increased heart rate). Vecuronium has even fewer side effects. Atracurium is hydrolysed spontaneously in the plasma and is therefore relatively safe and short-lasting.

Finally, a number of toxins including the snake toxin $\alpha$-bungarotoxin (from the krait, *Bungarus*) and najatoxin (from the cobra, *Naja*), bind irreversibly to nicotinic receptors at the neuromuscular junction. They produce a non-depolarizing block of transmission but are non-competitive.

### Depolarizing drugs

The second type of muscle relaxant drug initially and transiently mimics the effect of ACh, producing a depolarization of the end-plate. This sometimes causes an initial twitching of the muscle (which can result in a dangerous release of potassium) and subsequent muscle pains. One of the first synthetic depolarizing neuromuscular blocking drugs was **decamethonium** (C10, Figure 2.1), but only one such drug is used frequently in medicine—**suxamethonium** (**succinylcholine**). Whereas ACh is hydrolysed very rapidly, suxamethonium is hydrolysed much more slowly by cholinesterases, mainly by butyryl-cholinesterase in plasma. It can therefore remain active at the receptor for long periods (up to 7 minutes), producing a maintained depolarization of the end-plate. This leads to inactivation of voltage-operated sodium channels and thus failure to produce action potentials and contraction.

The short duration of action of suxamethonium means that the degree of muscle relaxation can normally be well and safely controlled by means of a continuous intravenous infusion. Some subjects have a heriditary lack or abnormality of plasma cholinesterase with the result that suxamethonium is not as rapidly metabolized. In these people the normally brief action of succinylcholine may last for hours and the normal dose of the drug may even prove life-threatening. Anaesthetists now test for the level of butyryl-cholinesterase in blood before using suxamethonium in patients. **Nicotine** (Figure 2.1), the tobacco constituent found to activate neuromuscular receptors and originating the description nicotinic, also acts in this way producing initial stimulation and subsequent blockade of neuromuscular transmission.

### Dual block

The blockade of ACh receptors by suxamethonium is essentially non-competitive. In the case of an overdose, therefore, increasing the concentration of ACh will not usually help the situation, and may make it worse by producing an even greater and longer lasting depolarization. However, the continued presence of the drug causes a change in the ACh receptors to a desensitized state which is less than normally responsive to agonists (ACh or drug). This results in a partial recovery of the membrane potential which in turn means that an increase in the local concentration of ACh can cause some weak muscle contraction; i.e. block can be partially reversed by, for example, anti-cholinesterases. The initial depolarizing block and the subsequent reversible block are sometimes known as Phase 1 and Phase 2 blockade respectively. Of course, the administration of a non-depolarizing blocking drug before a depolarizing blocking drug would reduce the effects of the latter by preventing association with the receptor.

# Acetylcholinesterases

Acetylcholinesterase (AChE) is a tetrameric protein complex with a molecular size of approximately 250 kDa. The mechanism by which the enzyme hydrolyses ACh is quite well understood from studies in which changes in the molecular structure have yielded changes in the efficiency of the hydrolysis. The sequence is summarized in Figure 2.3, which shows the presence of sites on the enzyme capable of binding the cationic head of ACh (the anionic receptor site) and the ester portion of ACh (the esteratic receptor site). After binding the whole ACh molecule the enzyme first splits it to free choline, leaving itself acetylated. The acetyl group is then hydrolysed from the enzyme to yield free acetate. One molecule of AChE is able to hydrolyse around 10,000 molecules of ACh each second.

## Anticholinesterases

Several drugs are available which inhibit the enzyme AChE and are therefore known as **anticholinesterases**. By preventing the rapid hydrolysis of ACh these drugs facilitate neuromuscular transmission by enhancing the degree and duration of end-plate depolarization. They are valuable drugs for reversing the effects of the non-depolarizing muscle relaxants such as tubocurarine after poisoning or surgery since the increased ACh concentration will compete with and displace the antagonist.

Anticholinesterases are also used in the disease of myasthenia gravis which is an autoimmune disease in which antibodies produced by the body itself interfere with the normal nicotinic ACh receptors, reducing end-plate responses to ACh. Sufferers therefore experience muscular weakness and may, without treatment, eventually need mechanical assistance to breathe. Cholinesterase inhibitors such as **neostigmine** or **physostigmine** (**eserine**) (Figure 2.1) provide

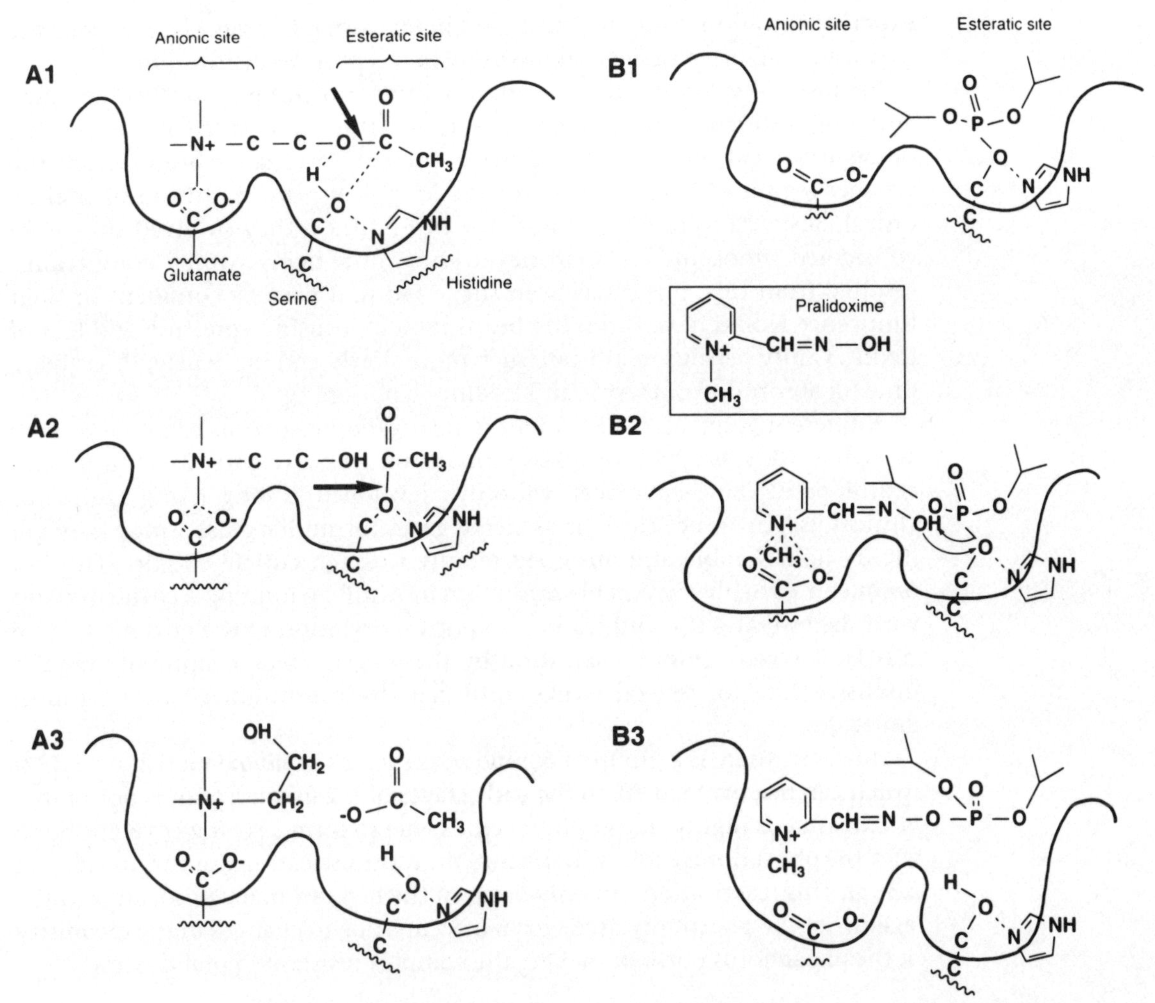


**Fig. 2.3** (A) Hydrolysis of acetylcholine by acetylcholinesterase (B) Illustrates the manner in which an organophosphorus anticholinesterase (dyflos, DFP) combines with acetylcholinesterase, and the way in which pralidoxine can combine with DFP so as to reactivate the enzyme and prevent irreversible inhibition.

some relief and improved neuromuscular function. A short-acting anticholinesterase, **edrophonium**, is used clinically as a diagnostic test for myasthenia gravis. It binds only to the anionic site of the enzyme and the bond formed is rapidly hydrolysed, giving the drug a duration of action of only a minute or two. Its ability to provide transient relief from muscular weakness is generally taken to be diagnostic of myasthenia gravis. Other cholinesterase inhibitors such as neostigmine (Figure 2.1) contain a carbamyl group which is much more slowly removed from the esteratic site of the enzyme than is the acetyl grouping of acetylcholine itself. The main difficulty of using anticholinesterase drugs is that they will also potentiate the effects of ACh at autonomic synapses (Chapter 3) leading to excessive salivation, mydriasis, exocrine secretion, bronchospasm and bradycardia. Conversely, frequent use may lead to reduced tissue responses due to receptor desensitization.

Because physostigmine is a non-quaternary compound (unlike most anticholinesterases), it also has effects on the brain since it crosses the blood–brain barrier. Indeed, eserine is present in Calabar beans (from the Calabar region of Nigeria), which have long been used in a form of trial by ordeal. Suspects were forced to eat the beans and if they survived they were considered innocent. We shall never know how many wrong 'convictions' resulted from this, but it has been suggested that persons confident in their innocence would have eaten the beans rapidly, causing vomiting and loss of toxins. Guilty persons might eat much more slowly and cautiously, thus giving time for absorption of eserine and leading to poisoning.

A different group of AChE inhibitors are organophosphorus compounds such as **dyflos** (diisopropylfluorophosphonate or DFP), (Figure 2.1), sarin and ecothiopate. These have been variously developed as long-acting agents for clinical use, as insecticides or as nerve gases for military use, since they are highly lipid soluble and absorbed rapidly through cuticle or skin. They all produce a virtually irreversible inhibition of AChE by forming a covalent bond with the esteratic site and leading to phosphorylation of the enzyme (Figure 2.3B1). Recovery from intoxication by these agents would normally require intensive care for several weeks until cells have synthesized new receptor molecules.

However, there is a group of compounds such as **pralidoxime** (Figure 2.3B2) which can reactivate AChE in the early stages of organophosphorus poisoning. Pralidoxime is highly nucleophilic and is able to form a strong covalent bond with the phosphorus moiety of the inhibitor, thus releasing the enzyme (Figure 2.3B3). This reactivation can only occur in the first few hours or so, after which 'ageing' of the phosphorylated enzyme occurs, due to changes in the chemistry of the phosphorus portion, making the complex resistant to pralidoxime.

# 3 The autonomic nervous system

## Introduction

The autonomic nervous system controls the activity of visceral structures—the smooth muscles, cardiac muscle and glandular secretions—over which we usually have little or no direct voluntary control. It is usually classified functionally or anatomically into sympathetic and parasympathetic systems and, since the parasympathetic system uses acetylcholine as its neurotransmitter, this will be considered first. An alternative method of classifying autonomic nerves is as cholinergic (using acetylcholine as transmitter), adrenergic (using noradrenaline/norepinephrine (NA/NE)* as transmitter) and non-adrenergic, non-cholinergic (NANC).

## The parasympathetic nervous system

The parasympathetic nervous system consists of nerves which originate either from the brain (the cranial nerves III (oculomotor); VII, (facial); IX (glossopharyngeal); and X (vagus), or from the sacral region of the spinal cord. The organs innervated and the major effects produced by the nerves are summarized in Figure 3.1. The axons travel from the central nervous system (CNS) to the various organs indicated, but they do not form synapses directly on the target cells. Instead they normally synapse onto a second set of nerve cells whose cell bodies are located in or close to the target tissue (Figure 3.2). These synaptic regions are known as ganglia, the neurons projecting to them from the CNS consequently being **pre-ganglionic** neurons and the cells projecting from a ganglion onto the visceral tissue being the **postganglionic** neurons (see Figure 3.2). The postganglionic cells form synapses onto the smooth muscle or

*NA/NE. A small problem which always arises in writing for an international audience is that of catecholamine nomenclature. The catecholamines known in the UK and many other countries as **adrenaline** and **noradrenaline** are known in the USA as **epinephrine** and **norepinephrine** respectively. In order to try and minimize the confusion this difference can cause I have used the joint abbreviations AD/E (adrenaline or epinephrine) and NA/NE (noradrenaline or norepinephrine) in this volume. Since the related terms adrenergic and adrenoceptors are universal (derived from adrenaline) they present no problem.

I have also introduced the abbreviation ISO to refer to the compound variously known in different countries as isopropylnoradrenaline, isopropylnorepinephrine, isoprenaline or isoproterenol.

Tissues innervated

Responses to nerves or muscarinic agonists

CRANIAL OUTFLOW

| Tissues innervated | Nerve | Responses to nerves or muscarinic agonists |
|---|---|---|
| Eye | III | contraction of ciliary m. (accommod.)<br>contraction of iris sphincter (miosis) |
| Lachrymal glands | VII | tear production |
| Salivary glands | IX | salivary secretion |
| Heart | X (Vagus) | ⬇ rate, atrial force, AV conduction |
| Respiratory system | X (Vagus) | bronchoconstriction; mucus production |
| Stomach | X (Vagus) | smooth muscle contractions;<br>parietal cell secretion |
| Small intestine | X (Vagus) | smooth muscle contraction;<br>⬆ motility & peristalsis; sphincter relaxation<br>exocrine secretion |

SACRAL OUTFLOW

| Tissues innervated | Responses to nerves or muscarinic agonists |
|---|---|
| Bladder | contraction of body (detrusor m.)<br>relaxation of sphincter |
| Large intestine | as for small intestine |
| Uterus | contraction in some species |
| Genitalia | dilation of blood vessels |

Pelvic nerves

Sacral cord

**Fig. 3.1** A summary of the parasympathetic nervous system, indicating the distribution (left) and functional effects (right) of the cranial outflow (cranial nerves III, VII, IX and X) and the sacral outflow.

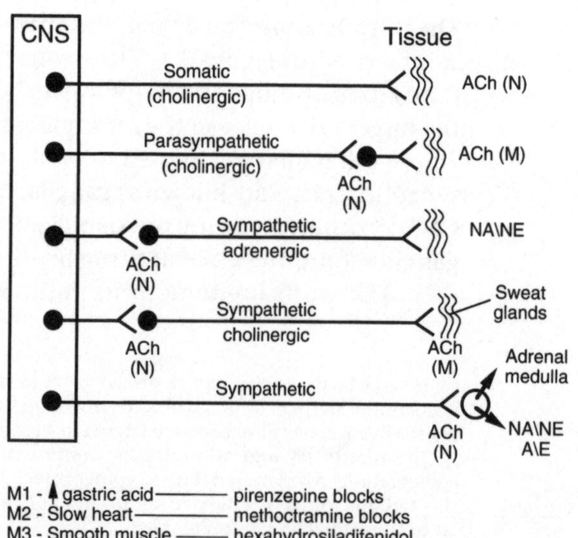


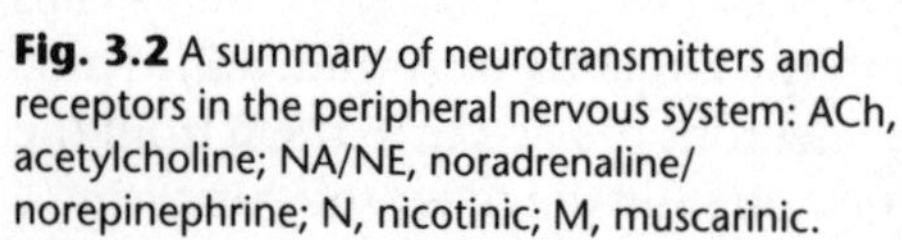

**Fig. 3.2** A summary of neurotransmitters and receptors in the peripheral nervous system: ACh, acetylcholine; NA/NE, noradrenaline/norepinephrine; N, nicotinic; M, muscarinic.

secretory tissue of visceral organs, these synapses being known as **neuroeffector junctions** (in contrast to the somatic, or skeletal neuromuscular junction, Chapter 2).

## Ganglionic receptors

In the parasympathetic nervous system, both pre- and postganglionic neurons release acetylcholine as their neurotransmitter, but there are important differences between the receptors for acetylcholine in the autonomic structures and those at the skeletal neuromuscular junction. The major receptors on the postganglionic neurons are, like the skeletal muscle receptors, activated and then blocked by nicotine (depolarizing block) and they are also therefore **nicotinic** receptors. However, d-tubocurarine and decamethonium are less active at blocking these ganglionic receptors than the neuromuscular variety, whereas shorter chain analogues of decamethonium, such as **hexamethonium**, are effective non-depolarizing blockers of ganglionic transmission which work by blocking the receptor-operated channel rather than the receptors themselves. Hexamethonium (C6) has little effect at the neuromuscular junction and the structure–activity relationships for the two sites are quite different (Figure 3.3).

There are also structurally unrelated agents which clearly discriminate between the two sites: the snake toxin, $\alpha$-**bungarotoxin**, blocks neuromuscular but non-ganglionic synapses and drugs such as **mecamylamine** (Figure 3.4) block only the ganglionic synapses. Trimethylammonium and dimethylphenylpiperazinium (DMPP) ions are acetylcholine-like (cholinomimetic) agonists at ganglionic nicotinic receptors. Ganglionic nicotinic receptors mediate fast synaptic transmission, with postsynaptic potentials lasting only a few milliseconds.

In addition, postganglionic neurons possess muscarinic receptors, similar to those described in the next section, which mediate a slow EPSP. The depolarization is due to the inhibition of a potassium current called the M

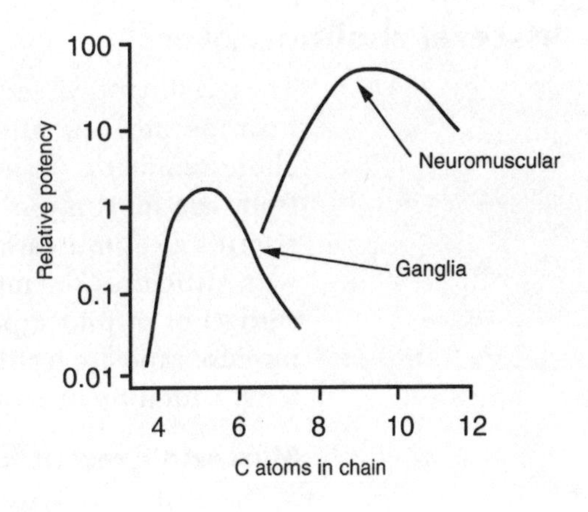


**Fig. 3.3** A graph showing the relationship between relative potency as acetylcholine antagonists and carbon chain length for a series of compounds. Maximum antagonist potency is seen at different molecular sizes for neuromuscular and ganglionic nicotinic receptors.

Decamethonium (C10) $(CH_3)_3 N^+ . (CH_2)_{10} . N^+ (CH_3)_3$
Hexamethonium (C6) $(CH_3)_3 N^+ . (CH_2)_6 . N^+ (CH_3)_3$

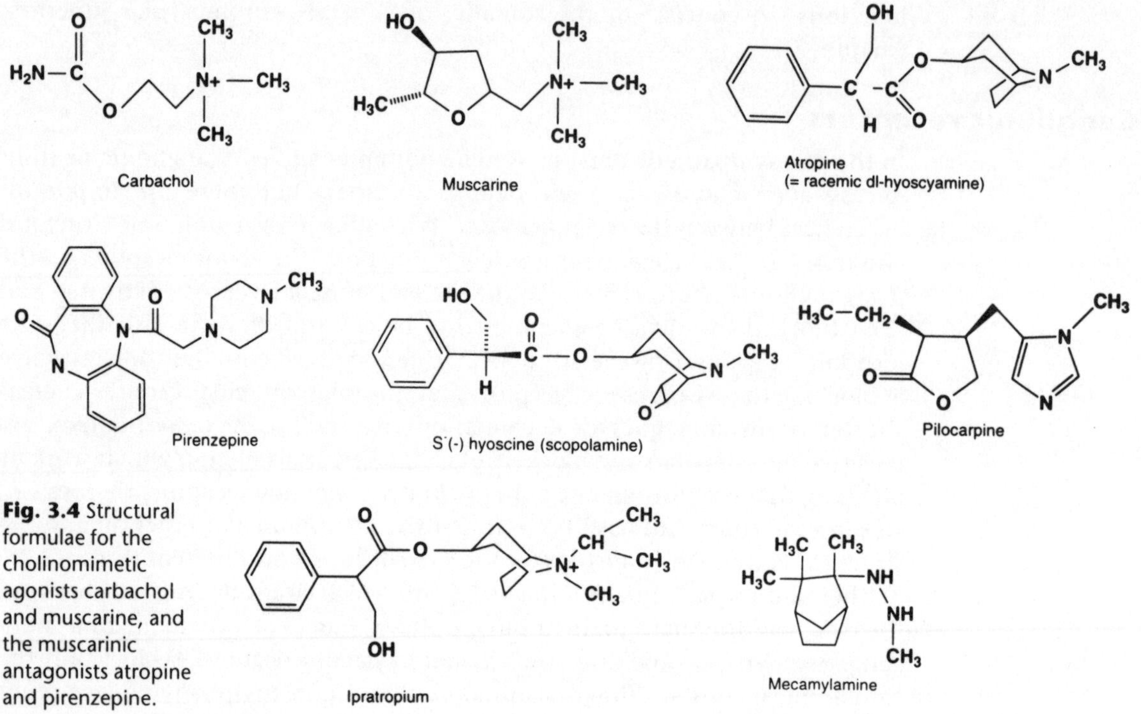

Carbachol

Muscarine

Atropine
(= racemic dl-hyoscyamine)

Pirenzepine

S(-) hyoscine (scopolamine)

Pilocarpine

Ipratropium

Mecamylamine

**Fig. 3.4** Structural formulae for the cholinomimetic agonists carbachol and muscarine, and the muscarinic antagonists atropine and pirenzepine.

current ($I_M$). Closure of these channels by cholinomimetics and some peptides such as substance P leads to depolarization which can modulate excitability for several seconds. There is also evidence for an IPSP produced by catecholamines released from cells within the ganglion, and a late, slow EPSP produced by a peptide, probably luteinizing hormone releasing factor, in some species.

## Visceral cholinoceptors

The receptor on visceral tissues for acetylcholine released by the postganglionic neurons are not affected by nicotine, but can be activated by another cholinomimetic (mimicking ACh) alkaloid **muscarine** (Figure 3.4), obtained from the mushroom *Amanita muscaria*. These cholinoceptors are therefore referred to as **muscarinic**. They may be stimulated by a number of substances with structures resembling acetylcholine (Figure 2.1), such as **methacholine**, **carbachol** or **pilocarpine** (Figure 3.4). These have little activity at nicotinic receptors and are relatively resistant to acetylcholinesterase, exhibiting a much longer duration of action than acetylcholine itself.

### Muscarinic receptor subtypes

At present it is possible to distinguish pharmacologically between three subtypes of muscarinic receptor, some properties of which are summarized in Table 3.1. All are G-protein coupled receptors with seven transmembrane-

**Table 3.1** Properties of muscarinic receptors

| Receptor (gene) | Sample location | Sample effect | G-protein | Transduction system | Selective antagonist |
|---|---|---|---|---|---|
| M1 (m1) | Brain: cortex, striatum, hippocampus | Depolarization | $G_q$ or $G_i/G_o$ | 1. Activation of phospholipase C | Pirenzepine |
| | Stomach | Acid secretion | | 2. Inhibition of M current ($I_M$) | |
| M2 (m2) | Heart; brain: cortex; spinal cord | Presynaptic inhibition of transmitter release | $G_i/G_o$ | 1. Inhibition of adenylate cyclase 2. Increase of potassium conductance | Methoctramine |
| M3 (m3) | Endocrine tissues; smooth muscle | Secretion; contraction | $G_q$ or $G_i/G_o$ | Activation of phospholipase C | Hexahydrosiladifenidol |
| | Brain: hippocampus | Depolarization | $G_q$ or $G_i/G_o$ | 1. Activation of PLC 2. Increase of cation conductances | |
| | Blood vessels | Formation of nitric oxide leading to relaxation | | NO causes activation of guanylate cyclase | |

spanning segments (Chapter 1). As a result, muscarinic effects are much slower than nicotinic responses, which are usually very transient and completed in a few milliseconds (either at skeletal or ganglionic sites). The inhibitory effect of muscarinic agonists on heart rate results from an increase of $gK^+$ which hyperpolarizes cells of the sinoatrial node and the atrioventricular conducting tissue. The receptor is coupled to the channel via a G-protein.

In some cases muscarinic receptors induce the formation and release of nitric oxide (NO) which in turn can stimulate guanylate cyclase. The resulting elevation of cyclic GMP levels may inhibit calcium fluxes and release and activate cyclic GMP-dependent protein kinase which in turn phosphorylates proteins. The final result is the dephosphorylation of myosin and relaxation of, for example, vascular smooth muscle. Gene cloning techniques have isolated five closely related genes (m1 to m5) so that at least two other subtypes of receptor may remain to be identified.

## Effects of muscarinic receptor stimulation

The pharmacological effects of stimulating muscarinic receptors on the visceral organs are generally those of activating the parasympathetic nervous system itself, as summarized in Figure 3.1. Note that most blood vessels do not receive any parasympathetic innervation but many do possess muscarinic receptors which induce relaxation of the vascular smooth muscle in response to locally produced or circulating cholinomimetics. The administration of acetylcholine and muscarinic agonists can therefore cause a profound and potentially hazardous fall of blood pressure. It was noticed around 1978 that segments of blood vessels removed from animals and tested *in vitro* often did not relax in response to added acetylcholine. Sensitivity seemed to depend on the manner of preparation. It was soon realized that vessels responded only if prepared with such extreme care that their delicate internal lining of endothelial cells was not damaged. If it was, acetylcholine had no effect. It was therefore proposed that acetylcholine acted on muscarinic receptors on the endothelial cells to trigger the release of an endothelial derived relaxant factor (EDRF) which subsequently diffused to the smooth muscle and caused relaxation. EDRF has now been identified as **nitric oxide** (NO).

### Clinical uses

Muscarinic agonists are used clinically to improve gastrointestinal motility and bladder function in neurological disorders where parasympathetic outflow has been affected, or following abdominal surgery when the intestine tends to be atonic and sluggish. A major use of these drugs is in the treatment of glaucoma. Aqueous humor in the anterior chamber of the eye is continuously secreted from epithelial cells and excess drains out through the canal of Schlemm near the outer perimeter of the iris. Obstruction of this drainage pathway can lead to elevated intraocular pressure (glaucoma) and a danger of retinal damage and blindness either due to reduced blood flow or detachment. By contracting the ciliary muscle and to some extent the iris sphincter (circular) muscle with muscarinic agonists drainage is improved and intraocular pressure falls.

In parasympathetically innervated tissues acetylcholinesterase is responsible for the destruction of acetylcholine, as at the neuromuscular junction, although this enzyme seems to be much less important at ganglionic synapses. The anticholinesterase drugs described in Chapter 2 will thus tend to induce parasympathetic-like (parasympathomimetic) effects on visceral tissues. Anticholinesterases such as physostigmine make a suitable alternative to the use of direct acting cholinomimetic agonists in glaucoma. The organophosphorus compound ecothiopate is also used for this condition since it has an extremely long duration of action (about 2 days). All these drugs would be applied as eye drops by instillation into the conjunctival sac, thus minimizing the amount needed and substantially reducing the dangers of widespread side effects on other tissues.

## Antagonists

A number of compounds are available which selectively block muscarinic cholinoceptors. They include natural alkaloids such as **atropine** (Figure 3.4) from the deadly nightshade plant *Atropa belladonna* and **hyoscine** from *Hyoscyamus niger*, both of which can also penetrate the blood–brain barrier and induce blockade of cholinoceptors in the CNS. This can lead to excitation, hallucinations and coma (atropine) or sedation and forgetfulness (hyoscine).

They also depress the vomiting centres of the brain and related drugs are valuable in treating travel (motion) sickness. These and related antagonists block all effect of peripheral muscarinic receptor stimulation.

A structurally different compound, **pirenzepine** (Figure 3.4) was found to block those muscarinic receptors responsible for stimulating acid secretion in the stomach far more readily than receptors on other tissues. This led to the subdivision of muscarinic receptors into three classes as noted above and in Table 3.1.

### Clinical uses of antagonists

Before the advent of modern pure drugs, *Atropa belladonna* was smoked by asthmatic patients to help relieve the bronchoconstriction. In general, the biological effects of muscarinic antagonists will be to prevent the effects of parasympathetic activity, leading to reduced gastrointestinal motility and peristalsis, increased heart rate, dry mouth due to reduced salivation, blurred near vision due to the failure of ciliary muscle contraction and thus accommodation (cycloplegia) and photophobia due to dilatation of the pupil. In patients susceptible to glaucoma the pupillary dilatation may also impede drainage of the aqueous humor and initiate a dangerous rise of intraocular pressure.

Muscarine antagonists do, however, have some clinical value by: (a) reducing gut motility to control diarrhoea; (b) dilating the pupil for examination of the retina; (c) preventing dangerous bronchial secretions in asthma, bronchitis or during anaesthesia for surgery; (d) reducing the parasympathomimetic side effects of anticholinesterases used in myasthenia; and (e) inhibiting gastric acid secretion in cases of peptic ulcer (although antagonists at histamine H2 receptors are much more widely used). Quaternary derivatives such as *N*-methylatropine and ipratropium (Figure 3.4) are often preferred for some of these effects since, being highly charged molecules, they are unable to cross the blood–brain barrier and thus cannot produce effects on the CNS. Ipratropium is used chiefly as an aerosol in asthma. Muscarinic antagonists which do penetrate the CNS are of use in motion sickness.

Unfortunately a large number of drugs which are used for other purposes also possess the ability to block peripheral muscarinic receptors to some extent; many of the symptoms just described, such as dry mouth, blurred vision, faecal and urinary retention may be seen as side effects of, for example, the tricyclic antidepressant drugs (Chapter 5).

## Sympathetic nervous system

The second division of the autonomic nervous system is the sympathetic (Figures 3.2 and 3.5). The sympathetic neurons originate in the intermediolateral cell column of the thoracic and lumbar regions of the spinal cord (Figure 3.5). As in the case of the parasympathetic system there are preganglionic neurons which release acetylcholine as their transmitter onto post-

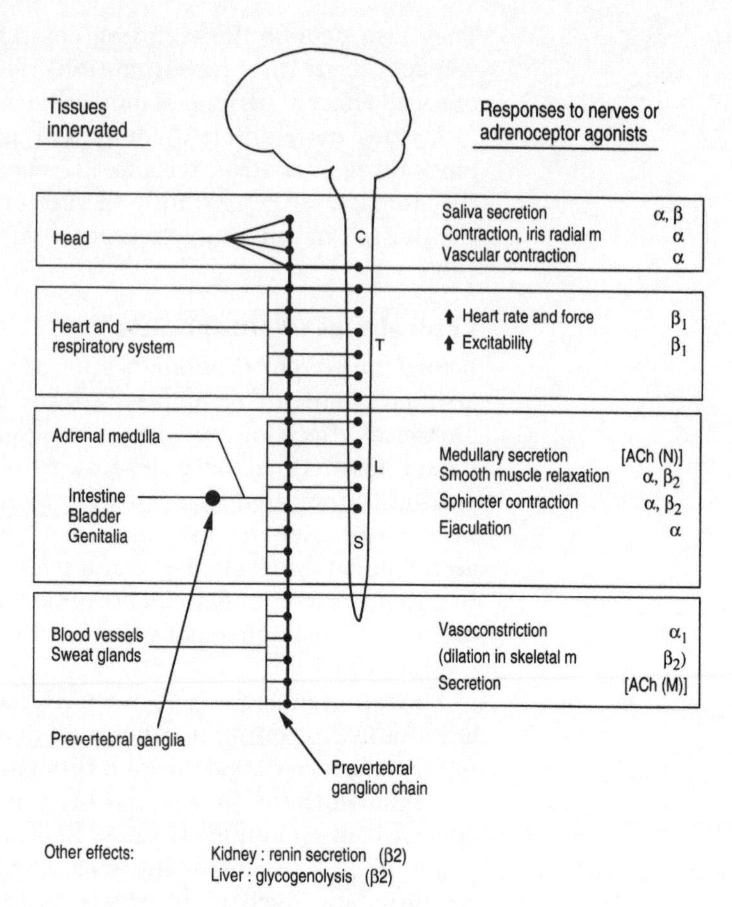


**Fig. 3.5** A summary of the sympathetic nervous system indicating the distribution (left) and functional effects (right) of the thoracolumbar outflow.

ganglionic cell bodies (Figure 3.2). In marked contrast to the parasympathetic nervous system however, the preganglionic axons are relatively short and the synapses are found mostly in two chains of ganglia, one on each side of the spinal cord, formed from ventral roots of the thoracolumbar outflow. These chains are known as the **paravertebral sympathetic ganglia**. The major fast transmission of information at the ganglia is mediated by cholinergic activation of ganglionic nicotinic receptors with essentially the same pharmacology as described above for the parasympathetic ganglia.

## Noradrenaline/norepinephrine (NA/NE)

At the endings of the postganglionic neuronal axons, making contact with the smooth muscle and secretory tissues of the viscera, the neurotransmitter is in most cases NA/NE (see footnote on page 23). The exceptions to this rule are that the postganglionic neurons causing secretion from sweat glands release acetylcholine as their transmitter as do some neurons innervating blood vessels in the face, skeletal muscle and external genitalia. The pharmacology here is identical with that of tissues innervated by postganglionic parasympathetic nerves (Figure 3.2).

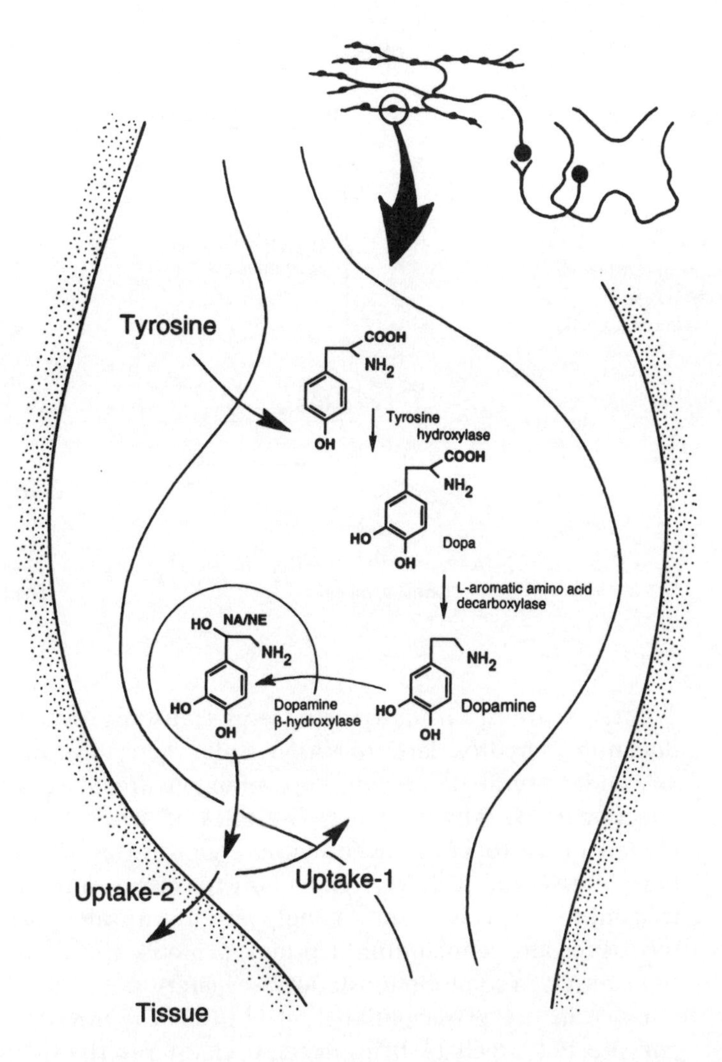


**Fig. 3.6** A diagram of the synthesis of NA/NE from tyrosine in sympathetic nerve terminals or varicosities.

A further peculiarity of the sympathetic nervous system is that it innervates the catecholamine secreting cells of the adrenal medulla, but the innervation is by preganglionic axons (Figures 3.2 and 3.5). The reason for this is that the medullary chromaffin cells have the same embryological origin as sympathetic postganglionic neurons. The chromaffin cells themselves thus release catecholamines and behave as postganglionic sympathetic neurons.

The structure of NA/NE is based on catechol and, like several other **catecholamines** is synthesized in nerve terminals from the amino acid tyrosine. The sequence of steps involved in this synthesis, and the enzymes responsible are summarized in Figure 3.6. Notice also from this diagram (and Figure 1.1B) that the sympathetic nerve endings do not usually form a close relationship with a clear subsynaptic membrane, as at the neuromuscular junction, but that the transmitter is synthesized in varicosities along the length of the axon terminal branches. These release transmitter NA/NE into a relatively large extracellular space.

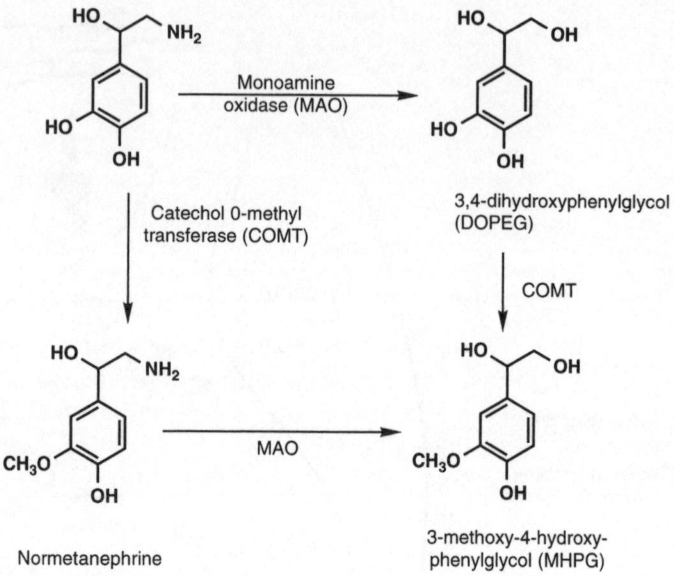

**Fig. 3.7** The metabolism of NA/NE via momoamine oxidase (MAO) and catechol-*O*-methyl transferase (COMT).

After synthesis from tyrosine and transport into the synaptic vesicles dopamine is hydroxylated to NA/NE and is then stored in the vesicle along with ATP and the synthetic enzyme dopamine $\beta$-hydroxylase. All these—NA/NE, ATP and dopamine-$\beta$-hydroxylase—are released when the vesicles release their contents (by exocytosis, as for cholinergic vesicles, Chapter 1). In many cases both NA/NE and ATP have effects on the tissue, and are then known as co-transmitters. This is an increasingly important principle in biology and many more substances, including peptides, proteins and lipids probably act as co-transmitters in some circumstances (see later).

Once in the extracellular fluid NA/NE is removed, not by a destructive enzyme, but largely by being taken back up into the sympathetic varicosities. This transport system is referred to as **Uptake 1** (Figure 3.6). There is also an Uptake 2 system which is a less important but high capacity transport system for NA/NE into non-neuronal cells such as smooth muscle and connective tissue. After being taken up NA/NE may suffer one of three fates. In non-neuronal tissue it is usually metabolized first by **catechol-*O*-methyltransferase** (COMT) (Figure 3.7) to inactive products and subsequently by **monoamine oxidase** (MAO). In the terminal varicosities it may either be transported back into vesicles or metabolized first by MAO, present on mitochondrial membranes, and then by COMT (Figure 3.7). The final product, easily detected in the urine, is 3-methoxy-4-hydroxyphenylglycol (MHPG).

## Drugs interfering with synthesis and storage

Several agents are available (Figure 3.8) which inhibit enzymes involved in the synthesis of NA/NE. These include **$\alpha$-methyl-*p*-tyrosine**, (which inhibits the rate-limiting synthetic enzyme tyrosine hydroxylase), **carbidopa** and **benserazide** (which inhibit L-aromatic amino acid decarboxylase, sometimes known as dopa decarboxylase). **Alpha-methyldopa** may also inhibit the latter enzyme to some extent although it is believed that this drug is mainly effective because it is metabolized to $\alpha$-methylNA/NE. This is less potent at $\alpha$-adrenoceptors than NA/NE itself and it thus has the effect of diluting the NA/NE stores and reducing the effects of sympathetic stimulation. Alpha-methylNA/NE is known as a false transmitter. Any of the above compounds may be used in situations where there appears to be an excessive activity of the sympathetic nervous system causing, for example, elevated blood pressure (hypertension). They are also of value in reducing catecholamine synthesis in tumours such as phaeochromocytoma (a tumour of adrenal medullary cells which can release massive amounts of catecholamines and cause serious hypertensive crises).

The natural alkaloid **reserpine**, the major active constituent in extracts of the plant *Rauwolfia*, prevents the transport and storage of catecholamines in synaptic vesicles. The vesicles thus initially release their amines and then rapidly become depleted of transmitter. **Tetrabenazine** has a similar action although its effects are reversible whereas those of reserpine are not.

## Drugs affecting release

Several powerful drugs act indirectly by displacing NA/NE from its storage vesicles, promoting its release and providing a sympathomimetic effect. They are known as **indirectly acting sympathomimetics**, and include **amphetamine**, **tyramine** and **ephedrine** (Figure 3.8), the central stimulation and euphoria produced by the first of these being the result of a marked effect on catecholamines in the CNS (Chapter 11). Amphetamine also inhibits Uptake 1 and repeated use can therefore lead to a depletion of amines from the terminals. Conversely several agents such as **guanethidine** are taken into the varicosities by Uptake 1 but they then inhibit the process of transmitter release. They are referred to as **adrenergic neuron blocking drugs**.

## Drugs affecting uptake

Uptake 2 can be inhibited by some steroids and NA/NE metabolites such as normetanephrine but these are of little practical importance. Many compounds are known which inhibit Uptake 1 and, by so doing, cause a substantial enhancement in the size and duration of tissue responses to released NA/NE. One of the oldest of these agents is **cocaine**, an alkaloid present in leaves of *Erythroxylon coca* which was used by South American natives to reduce fatigue and enhance the motivation for work (Chapter 11). Cocaine is a drug widely abused in modern society because of its stimulant actions on the CNS. However, its inhibition of Uptake 1 causes pronounced sympathomimetic effects including an increase of heart rate and blood pressure which can cause serious health problems if maintained or repeated. Other drugs such as **imipramine** and **amitriptyline** are also very effective inhibitors of amine uptake as will be discussed in detail in Chapter 5.

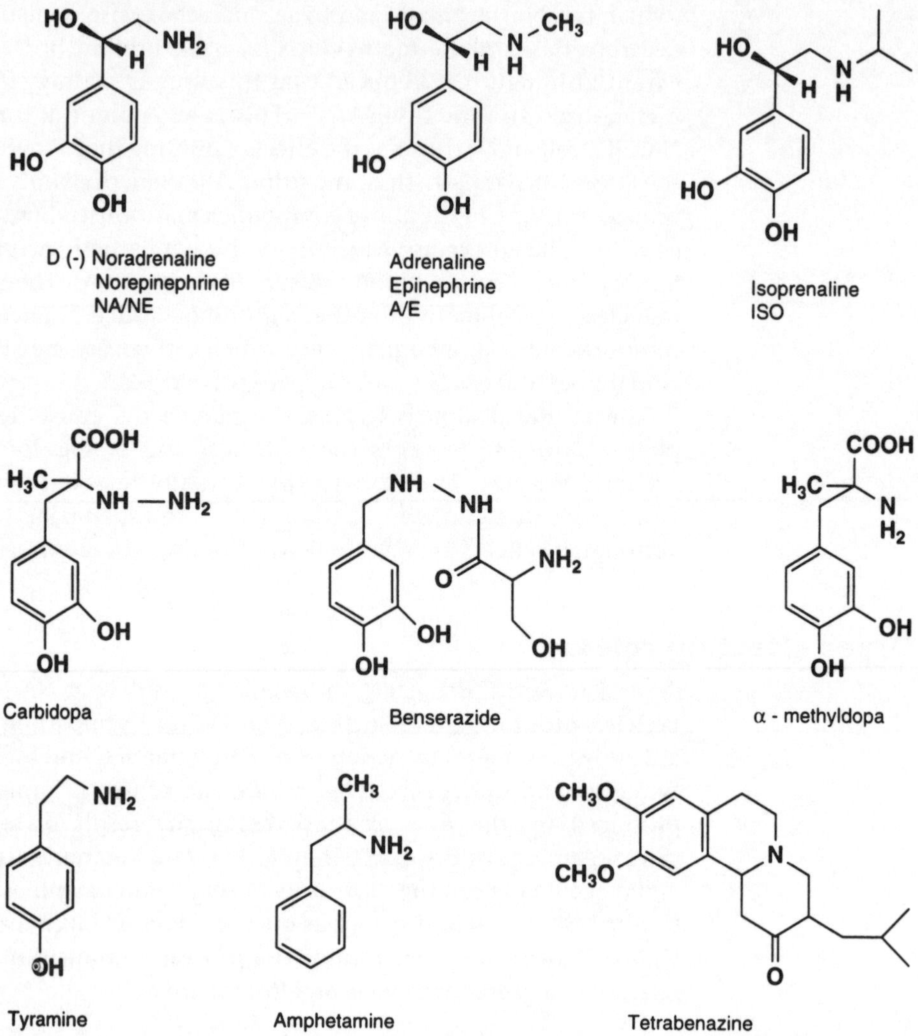

**Fig. 3.8** Structural formulae for NA/NE, AD/E and a variety of compounds acting upon the sympathetic nervous system.

D (-) Noradrenaline
Norepinephrine
NA/NE

Adrenaline
Epinephrine
A/E

Isoprenaline
ISO

Carbidopa

Benserazide

α - methyldopa

Tyramine

Amphetamine

Tetrabenazine

## Drugs affecting metabolism

The major enzyme involved in the destructive metabolism of NA/NE is monoamine oxidase (MAO). The major use of inhibitors of this enzyme is as antidepressants (Chapter 5) since by preventing the metabolism of NA/NE they are able to enhance the efficacy of adrenergic neuron activity. Because their actions are not confined to the CNS, there is a major problem of side effects due to overactivation of peripheral catecholamine receptors. This is a particularly dangerous problem if MAO inhibitors are present at the same time as indirectly acting sympathomimetics such as tyramine (present in some red wines, cheeses and beans). These amines are normally metabolized by MAO and if their metabolism, together with that of NA/NE are simultaneously inhibited the resulting overstimulation of receptors can cause a massive increase of blood pressure sufficient to cause vascular damage, haemorrhaging and death from internal bleeding or stroke.

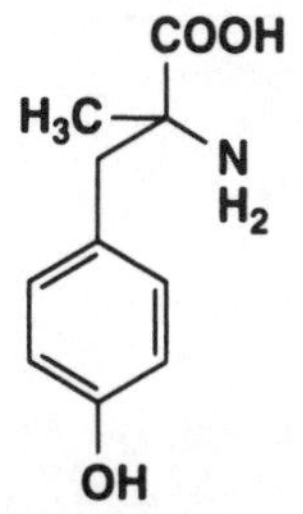

α - methyl-p-tyrosine

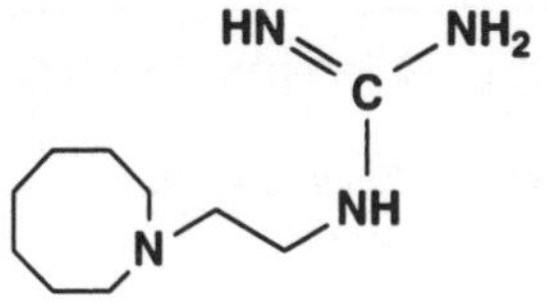

Guanethidine

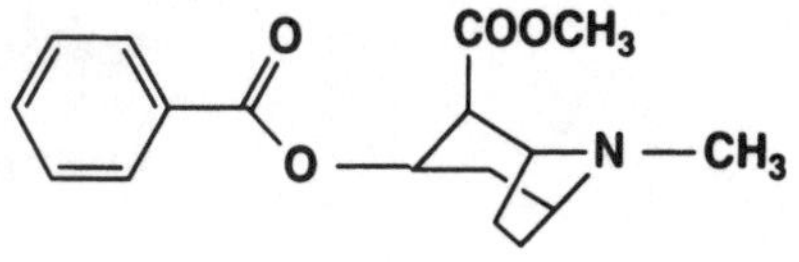

Cocaine

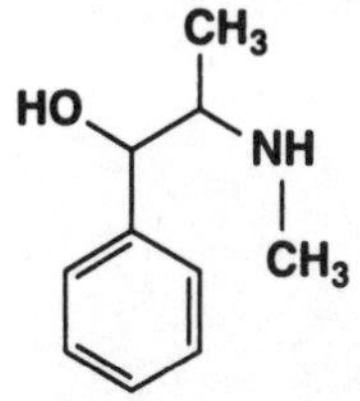

Ephedrine

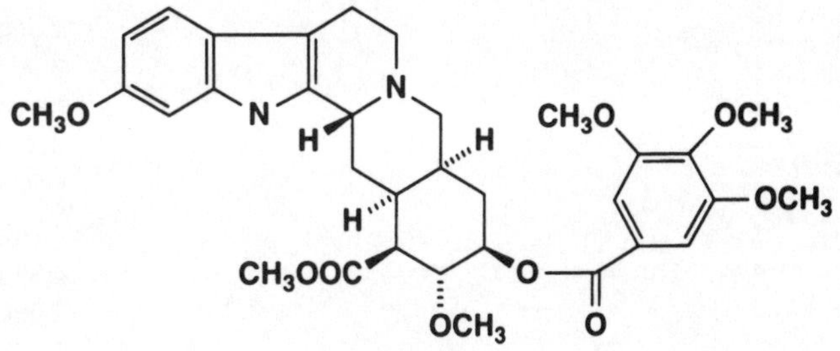

Reserpine

## Receptors for NA/NE

Ahlquist was among the first to record that several catecholamines had different potencies when eliciting sympathomimetic responses in the same tissues. **Adrenaline** (AD/E) (Figure 3.8) was more active than NA/NE in producing contraction of vascular muscle or radial muscle of the iris, and **isoprenaline** (isopropylNA/NE, isoproterenol, ISO) was less active than either. Conversely, ISO was the most active of these three agents and NA/NE the least active when causing stimulation of the heart or relaxation of vascular muscle. It was proposed that these differences might indicate the presence of different receptors responding differently to these and other catecholamines:

$\alpha$-receptors: AD/E > NA/NE > ISO

$\beta$-receptors: ISO > AD/E > NA/NE

In fact this classification has been extended further with the discovery that there are at least two types of $\alpha$ and two types of $\beta$ receptor, the properties of which are summarized in Table 3.2. All the NA/NE receptors are G-protein coupled and have the usual seven transmembrane-spanning segments as illustrated for the $\beta$-receptor in Figure 1.4.

The $\alpha$1-receptor is the form found mainly upon the smooth muscle and glandular cells and responsible for most of the excitatory and stimulatory actions of catecholamines. The main exception to this is that $\alpha$1-receptors cause relaxation of smooth muscle in the gut. The $\alpha$2-receptors have a much lesser effect on the smooth muscle itself, and are found mainly on nerve terminals as will be discussed later.

**Table 3.2** Properties of receptors for NA/NE

| Receptor | G-protein | Transduction system | Sample location and effect |
|---|---|---|---|
| $\alpha 1$ | $G_q$ | 1. Activation of phospholipases A2, C, D<br>2. Opening of L-type calcium channels | Smooth muscle contraction; (relaxation of intestine) |
| $\alpha 2$ | $G_i/G_o$ | 1. Inhibition of adenylate cyclase<br>2. Increase of $gK^+$<br>3. Activation of phospholipases A2, C<br>4. Closure of N-type calcium channels | Presynaptic inhibition of transmitter release; neuronal inhibition in CNS |
| $\beta 1$ | $G_s$ | 1. Stimulation of adenylate cyclase<br>2. Increase of calcium influx | Heart (increased rate and force) |
| $\beta 2$ | $G_s$ | | Bronchial smooth muscle (relaxation) |
| $\beta 3$ | $G_s$ | | Adipose tissue; lipolysis |

$\beta 1$-receptors occur almost exclusively on the heart where they cause an increased rate and force of contraction. (A similar receptor on fat cells promotes the metabolism of fat (lipolysis) but it is likely that this is a different subtype of receptor, $\beta 3$). $\beta 2$-Receptors mediate the relaxation of vascular and bronchial muscle and increase the availability of glucose by stimulating the breakdown of glycogen in the liver (glycogenolysis) and the synthesis of glucose from amino acids (gluconeogenesis). The nature of the receptors mediating these and other tissue responses to catecholamines are summarized in Figure 3.5.

The pattern of response to catecholamine receptor stimulation indicated in Figure 3.5 may at first appear complex, but some rationalization is possible when one recalls Canon's concept of the sympathetic nervous system as an emergency, or fright–fight–flight system. In the early days of human evolution (and in some parts of the world even now) an emergency system can mean the difference between death and survival. In such circumstances it seems sensible to:

- inhibit the muscle activity of immediately unimportant tissues (relaxation of stomach, intestine, bladder)
- close down blood supply to these and other unimportant tissues (vasoconstriction in gut and skin)
- increase blood supply to skeletal muscles (vasodilation)

- increase heart rate and thus blood pressure and muscle perfusion (cardiac stimulation).
- increase air supply (relaxation of tracheobronchial muscle)
- dilate the pupil (contraction of radial muscle; more light—important at night)
- increase the level of glucose for energy (glycogenolysis, gluconeogenesis)

All these changes are brought about when stressful situations result in the activation of sympathetic nerves, or release of AD/E from the adrenal glands.

## Chemical structure and biological activity

The large number of compounds available for studying catecholamine receptors have yielded much information on the relationships between molecular structure and receptor selectivity (Figure 3.9). Starting from AD/E for example it is known that:

(a) At least one ring hydroxyl is important for activity at any of the catecholamine receptors though many agents lacking these groups may still be able to act as indirectly acting sympathomimetics by releasing endogenous catecholamines (tyramine, ephedrine, amphetamine). Compounds with only one ring hydroxyl often lose $\beta$-receptor activity but can retain very strong $\alpha$-receptor stimulation (phenylephrine).

(b) The hydroxyl grouping on the $\beta$-carbon atom of AD/E is almost essential for significant stimulation of adrenoceptors. Dopamine, for example, is a very weak sympathomimetic. (There is a completely distinct set of receptors for amines such as dopamine on renal vessels, and in the CNS, as discussed in Chapter 4.)

(c) The insertion of a methyl group on the side chain $\alpha$-carbon increases activity at $\alpha$-receptors relative to $\beta$-receptors ($\alpha$-methyl-NA/NE, metaraminol)

(d) Increasing the size of the side chain, especially with substituents on the nitrogen atom increases the activity at $\beta$-receptors relative to $\alpha$-receptors (ISO, salbutamol, terbutaline).

(e) The two adjacent ring hydroxyls are essential for metabolism by COMT. Their separation or the intercalation of a methylene group yields compounds resistant to this enzyme (tyramine, salbutamol, terbutaline).

## Selective agonists and antagonists

Detailed structure–activity analyses of thousands of synthetic compounds and sophisticated computer-based analyses of molecular shape, size and conformation have been rewarded by the rational design of drugs with specific pharmacological properties and uses. For example, **salbutamol**, **terbutaline**, ritodrine and isoetharine are all drugs showing a strong preference for $\beta$2-

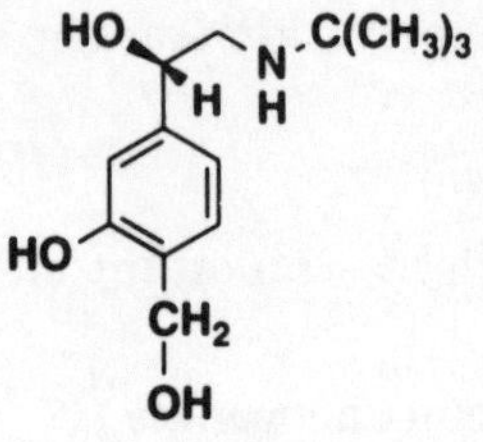

Salbutamol

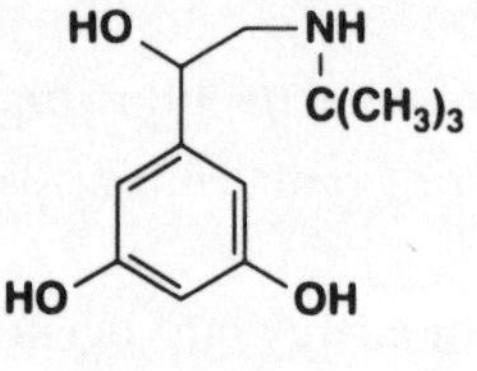

Terbutaline

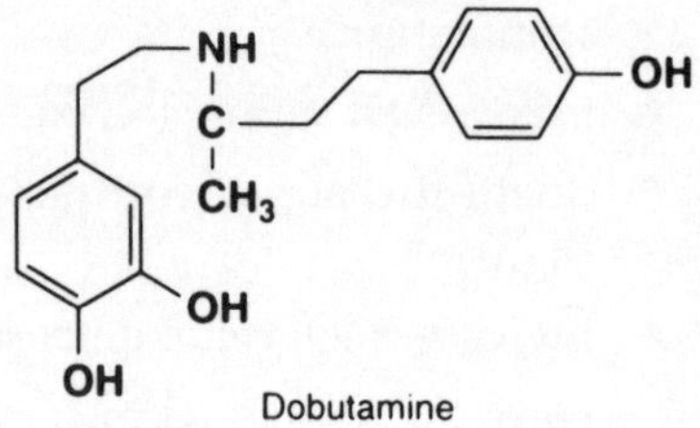

Dobutamine

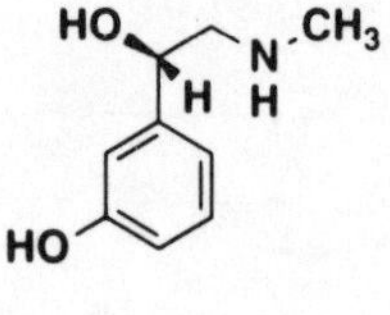

Phenylephrine

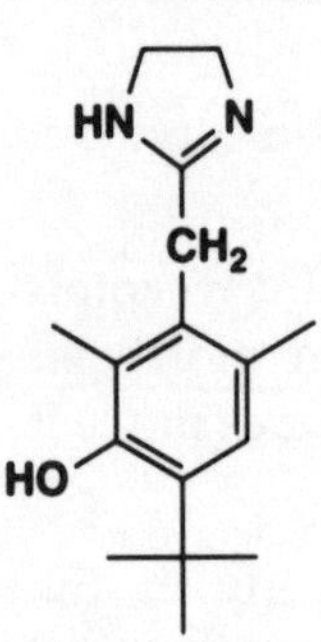

Oxymetazoline

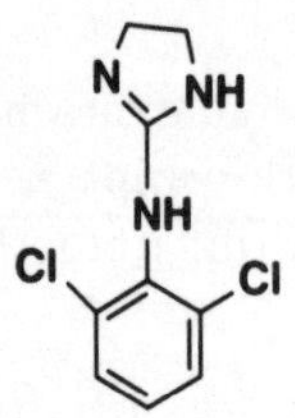

Clonidine

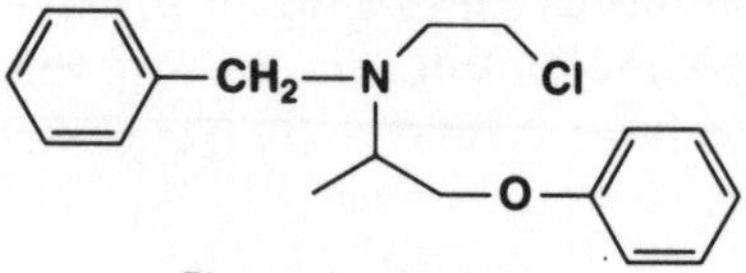

Phenoxybenzamine

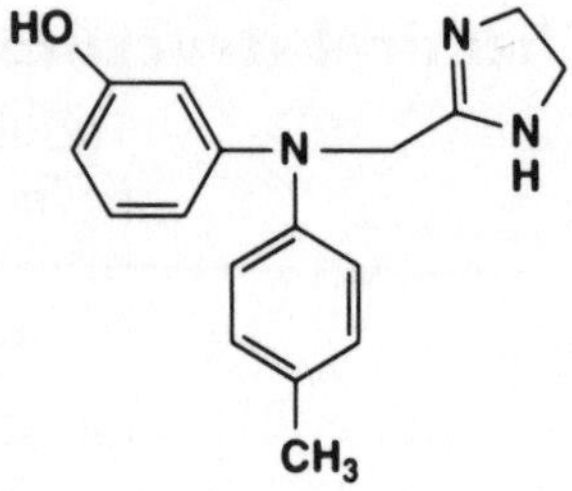

Phentolamine

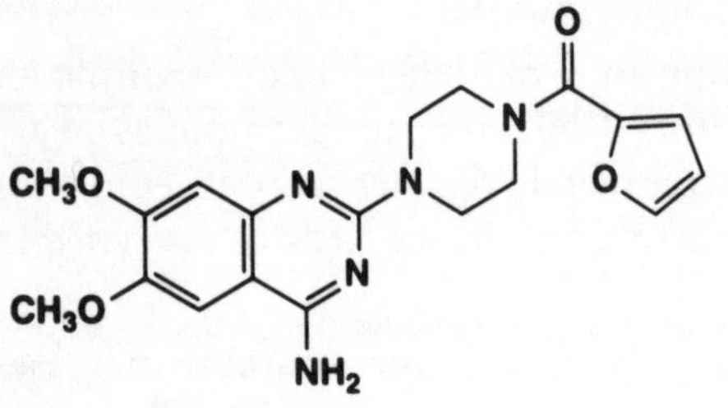

Prazosin

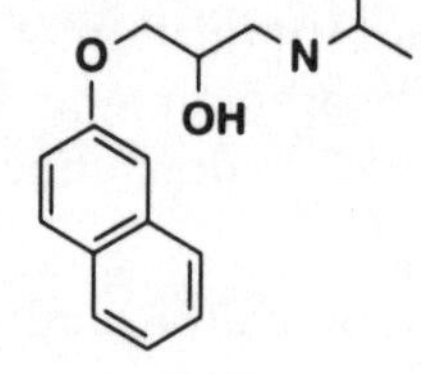

Propranolol

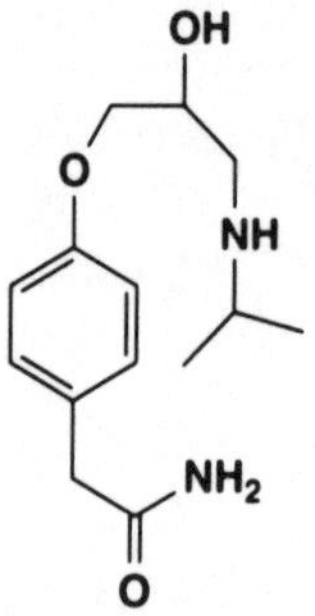

Atenolol

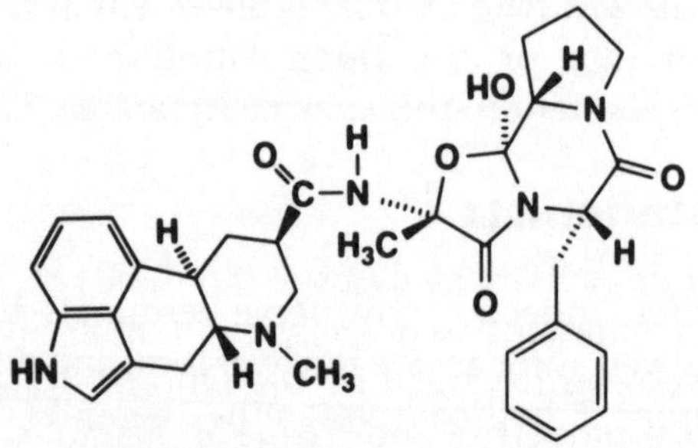

Dihydroergotamine

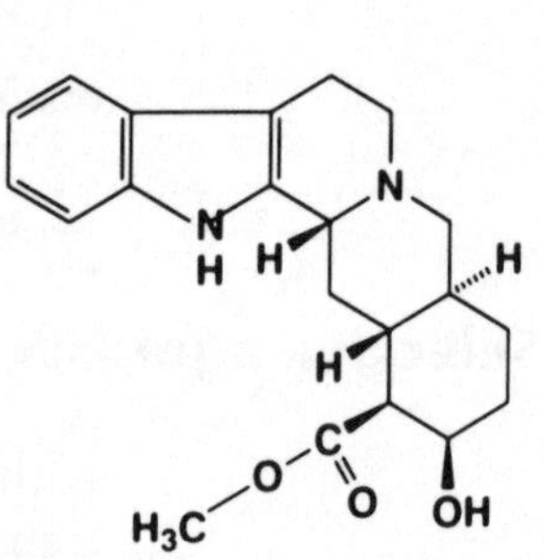

Yohimbine

**Fig. 3.9** Structural formulae for some sympathomimetic agonists and antagonists.

adrenoceptors. These drugs are used mainly for their ability to relax bronchial smooth muscle and thus prevent or abort asthmatic attacks. They carry the inestimable advantage over earlier, non-specific agonists such as AD/E or ISO in that they have virtually no stimulant action on the heart. The use of ISO in the treatment of asthma earlier this century resulted in several deaths due to accidental overstimulation of the heart. Terbutaline and ritodrine are used to inhibit uterine contractions and thus delay premature labour.

Conversely drugs such as **dobutamine** (Figure 3.9) have very high selectivity for $\beta 1$-receptors and thus find value as cardiac stimulants to increase the force, and to a lesser extent the rate, of contraction in cases of cardiac damage or failure.

Selective agonists are also available at $\alpha 1$-adrenoceptors (**phenylephrine**, **oxymetazoline**) and at $\alpha 2$-adrenoceptors (**clonidine**) (Figure 3.9). The former are used mainly as nasal decongestants. When sprayed or instilled locally they cause vasoconstriction in the nasal mucosa and thus inhibit nasal secretion, producing symptomatic relief from the common cold.

In order to understand the use and mechanism of action of clonidine, it is necessary to introduce the concept of presynaptic receptors.

## Presynaptic receptors

The discussion so far has concentrated on transmitter receptors located directly on smooth muscle or glandular cells, but receptors also occur on nerve terminals themselves. There is evidence for both cholinoceptors and adrenoceptors on motor nerve terminals at the neuromuscular junction, although presynaptic receptors are probably more important in the autonomic nervous system. On both cholinergic and adrenergic terminals there appear to be receptors for acetylcholine and NA/NE. The cholinoceptors on cholinergic terminals and adrenoceptors on adrenergic terminals are referred to as **autoreceptors** since the transmitter is in each case affecting its own release. The cholinoceptors on adrenergic terminals and adrenoceptors on cholinergic terminals are **heteroreceptors**.

The cholinergic autoreceptors are muscarinic (M2) and inhibit the release of acetylcholine. The adrenergic autoreceptors are of two types. The dominant one involves $\alpha 2$-adrenoceptors which inhibit the release of NA/NE. These receptors seem to function to prevent excessive release and thus potential depletion of transmitter when nerves are intensely active. There is also some evidence for presynaptic $\beta$-receptors which facilitate the release of the catecholamines.

The heteroreceptors, respectively muscarinic and $\alpha 2$ in nature, allow activity in one set of neurons to modify, or **modulate** the release of a different transmitter from other terminals. This is another important concept, that neurons and neurotransmitter systems do not work independently, but interact with each other. Indeed many nerve terminals bear receptors for several transmitters as well as for a wide range of local and distant hormones including amines (histamine, 5-hydroxytryptamine), peptides (kinins, opioids) and other agents (adenosine, ATP, prostaglandins, nitric oxide, etc.).

### $\alpha$2-Receptors

To return to $\alpha$2-receptors, it is this population of mainly presynaptic $\alpha$2-adrenoceptors for which clonidine is a reasonably selective agonist. Note, though, that clonidine does not have a catecholamine base structure, but is an imidazoline (Figure 3.9), a fact which emphasizes the different structural requirements of $\alpha$1- and $\alpha$2-receptors. At high doses clonidine can also activate $\alpha$1 sites.

The major use of clonidine therapeutically is in hypertension. By inhibiting the release of NA/NE from sympathetic nerve terminals clonidine reduces the degree of vasoconstriction and thus lowers peripheral resistance and systemic blood pressure. In fact this is only part of the explanation of clonidine's effect—most of it is mediated by a stimulation of $\alpha$2-receptors in the brain in areas which control sympathetic activity, the result being an overall reduction of sympathetic tone.

## Catecholamine antagonists

Structures of catecholamine antagonists are given in Figure 3.9. Some antagonists available for blocking adrenoceptors are given in Table 3.3. At the $\alpha$1-receptor, they include haloalkylamines such as **phenoxybenzamine**, which forms a covalent bond with the receptor molecule and induces a very long-lasting blockade, and **phentolamine**. There are also a number of alkaloids extracted from ergot (a fungus) such as **dihydroergotamine** which are partial agonists at $\alpha$-receptors and which are available for use in disorders which may involve excessive contraction of blood vessels in the hands (Raynaud's disease) or head (migraine). There are now far better drugs for migraine (Chapter 4). The non-selective $\alpha$-antagonists are also used to prevent the massive and dangerous activation of receptors which could otherwise result from the presence of catecholamine secreting tumours.

Selective antagonists are also available such as **prazosin** which blocks only $\alpha$1-receptors and thus reduces sympathetic tone and lowers blood pressure. Non-selective $\alpha$-antagonists cause some undesirable stimulation of heart rate and force owing to the blockade of presynaptic $\alpha$2-receptors (resulting in more NA/NE being released onto $\beta$-receptors). This is not a problem with selective $\alpha$1 antagonists.

**Yohimbine** and **rauwolscine** are selective antagonists at $\alpha$2-adrenoceptors. The latter is, like reserpine, an alkaloid from the *Rauwolfia* plant and it is interesting to note the similarity in structure between reserpine (Figure 3.8) and yohimbine (Figure 3.9).

The main problem with treating hypertension with $\alpha$-adrenoceptor antagonists is that reflex vasoconstriction (especially venoconstriction) in response to exercise or changes of posture are prevented as well as resting sympathetic tone. Such postural hypotension can cause dizziness and fainting, especially in the elderly. Visceral blood flow will also be increased and impotence or failure of ejaculation may occur due to blockade of the $\alpha$1 mediated sympathetic innervation to the vasa deferentia.

**Table 3.3** Drugs acting on noradrenergic neurons

| **Agonists** | **Receptors** | **Sample location** |
|---|---|---|
| NA/NE | $\alpha 1$, $\alpha 2$, $\beta$ | |
| Phenylephrine | $\alpha 1$ | Vascular smooth muscle |
| Clonidine | $\alpha 2$ | Presynaptic terminals; CNS |
| Isoprenaline (ISO) (isoproterenol) | $\beta 1$, $\beta 2$ | |
| Dobutamine | $\beta 1$ | Heart |
| Salbutamol | $\beta 2$ | Bronchi; liver |
| **Antagonists** | | |
| Prazosin | $\alpha 1$ | |
| Yohimbine | $\alpha 2$ | |
| Phentolamine | $\alpha 1$, $\alpha 2$ | |
| Propranolol | $\beta 1$, $\beta 2$ | |
| Atenolol | $\beta 1$ | |
| Metoprolol | $\beta 1$ | |
| Butoxamine | $\beta 2$ | |
| **Indirect sympathomimetics** | | |
| Amphetamine | | |
| Tyramine | | |
| Ephedrine | | |
| **False transmitters** | | |
| Metaraminol | | |
| $\alpha$-methyldopa | | |
| **Adrenergic neuron blockers** | | |
| Guanethidine | | |
| Bretylium | | |
| **Tyrosine hydroxylase inhibitors** | | |
| $\alpha$-methyl-*p*-tyrosine | | |
| **Monoamine oxidase inhibitors** | | |
| Pargyline | | |
| Iproniazid | | |
| Tranylcypromine | | |
| Clorgyline (MAO-A) | | |
| Deprenyl (selegiline) (MAO-B) | | |

It is important to emphasize that not all drugs acting at adrenoceptors are directly related to or derived from the catecholamine structure of AD/E. Several, for example, are imidazolines, including the $\alpha 1$ agonist oxymetazoline, the $\alpha 2$ agonist clonidine and the $\alpha 1/\alpha 2$ antagonist phentolamine.

Propranolol (Figure 3.9) is one of the most widely used antagonists at $\beta$-adrenoceptors (a '$\beta$-blocker'). It blocks both the $\beta 1$- and $\beta 2$-receptors. One of the major clinical uses of propranolol is in the treatment of hypertension. The mechanism of its hypotensive effect is not fully understood but probably results from a number of contributory actions such as:

- blocking the sympathetic drive to the heart, thus lowering heart rate and cardiac output
- blocking the facilitatory $\beta$-receptor on sympathetic nerve terminals, thus reducing NA/NE release
- blocking the sympathetic release of the enzyme renin from the kidney. Renin (pronounced reenin) is an enzyme which normally initiates splitting of angiotensinogen in the blood leading to the powerful vasoconstrictor angiotension II
- possible effects on the CNS to reduce sympathetic outflow

Compounds related to propranolol are also available, such as **alprenolol** and metoprolol, which are selective antagonists at $\beta 1$-receptors. By reducing the activity of the heart these compounds reduce the oxygen and vascular demand of this organ and are thus used to reduce angina. The selectivity of the $\beta 1$ blockade is important since they will not affect $\beta 2$-receptors in the bronchi. A blockade of $\beta 2$-receptors might initiate an asthmatic attack in susceptible persons.

## NANC nerves

In cases where neither acetylcholine nor NA/NE seem to be the transmitter of autonomic nerves, the neurons are referred to as NANC, or **non-adrenergic, non-cholinergic** nerves. They are present in both the sympathetic and parasympathetic nervous systems and include neurons releasing the purine nucleotide adenosine triphosphate (ATP) (purinergic nerves) and neurons releasing peptides such as substance P, vasoactive intestinal peptide, neuropeptide Y, cholecystokinin, somatostatin and several others (peptidergic nerves). The peptides are often stored in neurons in vesicles separate from those containing other transmitters such as ACh or NA/NE. There is some evidence that the release of amines and peptides can occur independently. When neurons are showing little activity they are able to preferentially release the amine transmitter. At high frequencies of stimulation, however, the peptide is also released. The dual release of a 'classical' neurotransmitter and a neuropeptide, or purine is known as **co-transmission**.

### Purines

Adenosine and adenosine triphosphate (ATP) are components of all cells, but both are released from cells into the extracellular medium, and both have marked effects on peripheral tissues and the CNS. ATP is stored together with ACh or NA/NE in their respective synaptic vesicles, and is released along with these transmitters from the synaptic terminals as a **co-transmitter**.

In the extracellular space, ATP is rapidly metabolized to adenosine by nucleotidase and ATPase enzymes. The effects of ATP are usually exerted on the postsynaptic cell, producing contraction or relaxation of smooth muscles. Adenosine, however, acts mainly on presynaptic inhibitory receptors to suppress neurotransmitter release. It can also act directly on vascular muscle to promote relaxation. For this reason it has been considered a compensatory or protective agent in tissues, having the dual actions of diminishing the release of stimulatory transmitters, and increasing blood flow and thus nutrient supply to active cells. In addition to having independent actions, ATP also potentiates the effects of NA/NE on some tissues.

The various receptors for adenosine and ATP are summarized in Table 3.4. The receptors for the adenine nucleosides such as adenosine are known collectively as P1 receptors. Receptors for adenine nucleotides such as ATP are known as P2 receptors.

### Substance P

Substance P is an 11 amino acid peptide. It is one of a group of peptides known collectively as **tachykinins**, and which includes neurokinins A and B. They are synthesized in neurons as the precursor protein preprotachykinins. The receptors for tachykinins are all G-protein linked (seven transmembrane regions) and all act via $G_q$ or $G_i/G_o$ to activate phospholipase C. There appear to be three subtypes of tachykinin receptors, the NK1 site responding best to substance P, the NK2 site responding best to neurokinin A, and the NK3 receptor responding best to neurokinin B.

**Table 3.4** Properties of purine receptors (adenosine and ATP)

| Receptor | Sample location | Sample effect | G-protein | Transduction system | Agonist | Antagonist |
|---|---|---|---|---|---|---|
| **P1 receptors (for adenosine)** | | | | | | |
| A1 | Presynaptic | Inhibition of transmitter release | G? | 1. Increase of $gK^+$ Decrease of $gCa^{++}$ | CPA | CPX |
| | | | $G_i/G_o$ | 2. Inhibition of adenylate cyclase | | |
| A2 | Vascular muscle | Relaxation | Gs | Stimulation of adenylate cyclase | DPMA | DMPX |
| A3 | Lungs | ? | ? | ? | – | – |
| **P2 receptors (for ATP)** | | | | | | |
| P2x | Smooth muscles: vas, intestine, bladder, blood vessels | Contraction | | Increase of cation conductances | $\beta\gamma$ mATP | – |
| P2y | Taenia coli, blood vessels | Relaxation | | Increase of potassium conductance | 2MeSATP | Reactive blue 2 |

The tachykinins cause contraction of smooth muscle in the intestine and may mediate the peristaltic response to gut stimulation seen during blockade of all ACh receptors. Substance P may also be responsible fo the cutaneous vasodilatation and increase of capillary permeability seen following a potentially injurious stimulus (the axon reflex). In ganglia, substance P can suppress the M current, leading to depolarization.

### Vasoactive intestinal peptide

Vasoactive intestinal peptide (VIP) is a 28 amino acid peptide originally discovered as a potent vasodilator in extracts of the intestine, but since recognized to occur in synaptic vesicles in a population of peripheral autonomic nerves. It can act upon two varieties of receptor, $VIP_1$ and $VIP_2$, both of which act via $G_s$-proteins to stimulate adenylate cyclase and increase cyclic AMP levels. VIP promotes exocrine secretions in the gut and is a powerful inhibitor of smooth muscle contraction. It relaxes many smooth muscles including the bronchi, and most blood vessels. It is present in cholinergic neurons innervating salivary and sweat glands. When neuronal activity is sufficiently intense, VIP is co-released with ACh. It then potentiates the secretory activity of ACh, but also induces a massive increase of local blood flow so that the rapidly secreting cells are kept amply supplied with oxygen and other nutrients.

### Neuropeptide Y

Neuropeptide Y is a 36 amino acid molecule which is present in many noradrenergic neurons such as those supplying the vas deferens and blood vessels. Once released, it acts upon two receptor subtypes, Y1 and Y2. Both of these are coupled by $G_i/G_o$ to inhibit adenylate cyclase, and the Y2 site can in addition act via a G-protein to close calcium channels. The peptide can potentiate the contractile effects of NA/NE, primarily via Y1 receptors. This is the predominant interaction seen at low levels of neuronal activity, when release is small. With more intense activity, the greater extracellular concentration of neuropeptide Y acts on presynaptic Y2 receptors and inhibits NA/NE release.

### Somatostatin

Somatostatin (SST) is sometimes known as somatotrophin (growth hormone) release inhibitory factor (SRIF). SST exists in two forms containing 14 and 28 amino acids (SST-14 and SST-28) both synthesized from preproSST. It is present in vesicles in neurons widely distributed around the body, particularly in the intestine. Here it causes marked inhibition of contractility. As it is released from the myenteric plexus of the gut upon distension, it is possible that SST-releasing neurons contribute to the reflex inhibition of the intestine. SST acts on at least two subtypes of receptors SST-1 (SRIF-1) and SST-2 (SRIF-2), both of which are G-protein linked with seven transmembrane segments. Each may exist in several forms (SST-1A-C; SST-2A-C) but all seem to inhibit adenylate cyclase and reduce calcium influx into cells.

### Nitric oxide

More recent additions to this group of neurotransmitters are nitric oxide (NO) and possibly carbon monoxide (CO). Nitric oxide is probably produced from the amino acid L-arginine and/or a nitrosothiol compound released from cells. Its synthesis can be blocked by inhibitors of nitric oxide synthase such as L-nitroarginine. Once released NO activates guanylate cyclase to produce smooth muscle relaxation or changes of neuronal excitability. Its ability to cause dilatation of blood vessels is the basis of the actions of nitrovasodilators such as glyceryl trinitrate, and is so powerful that it is now the candidate considered most likely to mediate the vasodilatation of blood vessels in the external genital organs.

# 4 CNS neurotransmitters

## Introduction

In order to assist the reader unfamiliar with neuroanatomy to orientate him/herself when reading this chapter, a summary diagram of the brain, indicating most of the areas mentioned, is given in Figure 4.1.

In addition, this figure summarizes the features of the **blood–brain barrier**. In peripheral vascular capillaries the lining endothelial cells are separated by gaps or 'fenestrations' through which proteins, white cells and drugs are relatively free to pass. In the brain, these spaces are absent, endothelial cells having 'tight junctions' between them which form a barrier to the passage of materials. Compounds can only enter the brain if : (a) they are lipid soluble and can

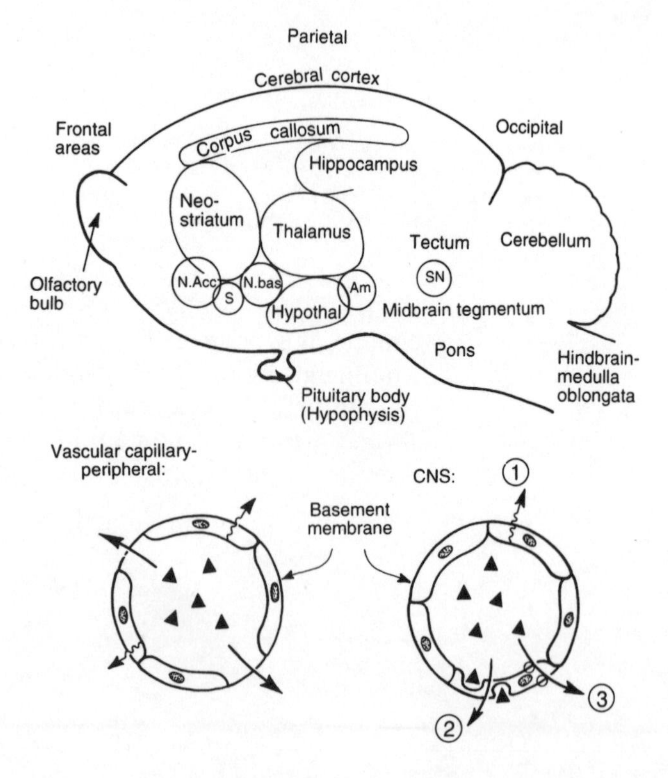


**Fig. 4.1** A diagram of the brain to show the location of major centres referred to in the text. The basis of the blood–brain barrier is illustrated. In peripheral vascular capillaries solutes can diffuse relatively freely into the tissues through gaps or fenestrations. In the CNS, adjacent endothelial cells are tightly coupled through 'tight junctions' and blood-borne compounds can only enter the brain by (1) being sufficiently lipid soluble to diffuse through the cell membranes, (2) being taken up and transported across the cell by endocytosis or (3) being a substrate for a transporter system such as those for amino acids or sugars.

diffuse through the cell membranes; (b) they are transported across the walls by specific enzymes (e.g. some amino acids); and (c) they are taken up into vesicles in the cells by endocytosis, being released later at the neuronal side of the capillary.

This is advantageous in the development of drugs for peripheral use, but presents major problems for drugs intended for CNS use. The structure of active molecules must often be modified to incorporate substituents which increase the lipophilicity, and thus access across the blood–brain barrier, without affecting the biological activity. This can be difficult.

# Neurotransmitters

In the CNS it can often be difficult or impossible to fulfil the various criteria listed in Chapter 1 for identifying a neurotransmitter. This is largely because of the presence of so many neurons releasing perhaps 50 or more different transmitters. In addition, interactions between transmitters are common. The adenosine A2 receptor for example reduces responses to the dopamine D2 receptor. Many compounds can also act upon presynaptic receptors to alter the release of themselves or other neuroactive agents, and the stimulation or inhibition of receptors can result in long-term changes of receptor number (up- or down-regulation). For these reasons a distinction is sometimes made between neurotransmitters and neuromodulators. The former would be released to produce primary effects of their own on neuronal activity. Neuromodulators would then be defined as compounds which have relatively little activity on their own, but which primarily modify the release of, or responses to, neurotransmitters. This distinction, however, is subtle and rather arbitrary, and should be viewed with caution. Most substances are best classified under the general term neuroactive compounds. In the following sections, some features of substances with clearly defined transmitter functions will be summarized.

## Acetylcholine

In the CNS acetylcholine (ACh) is synthesized from acetylcoenzyme A and choline, as in peripheral nerves, and choline is salvaged from the synaptic space. Cholinergic neurons can therefore be localized by staining with antibodies to the synthetic enzyme, choline acetyltransferase. This technique has revealed several major areas containing cholinergic cell bodies, and their projection pathways (Figure 4.2):

- neurons in the nucleus basalis (NB), or basal forebrain, (nucleus of Meynert) projecting to the cerebral cortex
- neurons in the septum (S) projecting to the neocortex and the hippocampus
- neurons in the pedunculopontine and lateral tegmental nuclei (PP/LT) projecting to the thalamus

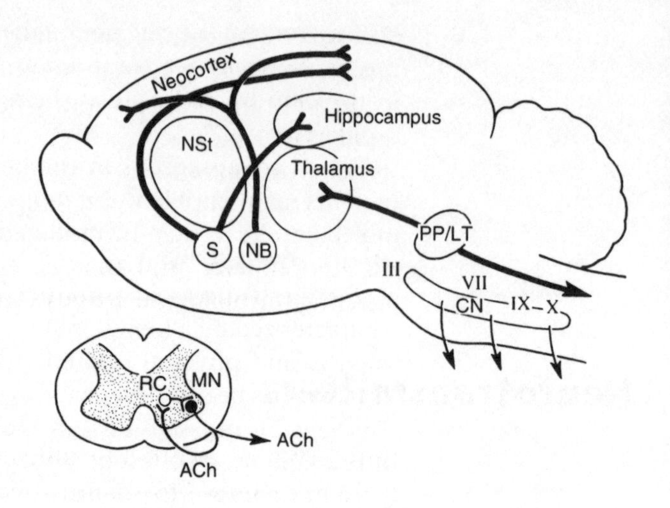


**Fig. 4.2** The major cholinergic projection pathways in the CNS. MN, motoneurones; RC, Renshaw cell; NSt, neostriatum; S, septum; NB, nucleus basalis, or ventrobasal complex; PP/LT, pedunculopontine nucleus and lateral tegmentum; III, VII, IX and X, cranial nerve outflow.

In addition, there are the preganglionic neurons of the parasympathetic cranial nerve nuclei III, VII, IX and X (CN in Figure 4.2), and small local cholinergic neurons in the neostriatum (NSt). In the spinal cord (inset, Figure 4.2) collateral branches of $\alpha$-motoneuron (MN) axons re-enter the cord to synapse onto inhibitory Renshaw cells (RC). The motoneuron transmitter is ACh, as it is peripherally; the Renshaw cell transmitter is the inhibitory amino acid glycine. As in peripheral tissues, ACh is released by depolarization from synaptic vesicles by calcium-dependent exocytosis, and is hydrolysed by an acetylcholinesterase.

### Receptors to acetylcholine

Both muscarinic and nicotinic cholinoceptors occur in the CNS, though relatively little is known about the nicotinic sites. They can be excited by nicotine and blocked by $\alpha$-bungarotoxin and usually induce depolarization of central neurons. Whereas the skeletal muscle receptors consist of two $\alpha$, one $\beta$, one $\gamma$ and one $\epsilon$ subunits (Chapter 1; Figure 1.5), the brain nicotinic receptors seem to be much simpler and consist only of $\alpha$ and $\beta$ subunits.

The muscarinic receptors can be classified pharmacologically into at least three subtypes—M1, M2, M3, as described in Chapter 3. Some receptor characteristics are summarized in Table 3.1. At M1 receptors ACh suppresses the voltage sensitive potassium current (M current) which is activated by membrane depolarization. This current normally serves to limit depolarization (enhancing spike accommodation). By suppressing this current ACh increases neuronal excitability.

At M2 receptors ACh usually increases a potassium conductance, resulting in hyperpolarization, and also reduces calcium conductances. M2 sites are often located on cholinergic cell bodies and synaptic terminals, functioning as presynaptic inhibitory receptors to reduce cell firing and diminish transmitter release. M3 receptor activation often causes an increased cation conductance and depolarization of neurons.

In addition, ACh induces a decrease of the calcium-dependent potassium current which causes afterhyperpolarization following an action potential. The receptor involved has not been clearly determined but has properties different from M1 and M2.

## Alzheimer's disease

Alzheimer's disease occurs in 10% of people over 65 years of age and is characterized by a loss of memory and mental confusion, progressing to total mental and physical disability. One of the most consistent neurochemical findings has been a degeneration of cholinergic cells in the nucleus basalis (NB, Figure 4.2) and septum (S). One of the main septal projection areas, the hippocampus, is believed to be important for learning and memory (damage to both hippocampi prevents learning) and the cholinergic projection to the hippocampus appears particularly important. Drugs which block muscarinic ACh receptors in the CNS (such as scopolamine) produce marked amnesia (and are used for this purpose during childbirth). Destruction of cholinergic neurons using the experimental compound ethylcholine aziridinium ion (AF64A) has a similar, though greater, effect. There is a great deal of research into the development of drugs which may maintain some cholinergic function and delay the symptoms of Alzheimer's disease—agents such as $\alpha$-glycerylphosphorylcholine which raises ACh release; nerve growth factor (NGF), which promotes growth of central cholinergic neurons; **eserine** (Figure 2.1) or **tetrahydroaminoacridine** (tacrine) which inhibit acetylcholinesterase; or M1 receptor agonists. These and other drugs which may increase mental function are known as cognitive enhancers or nootropic drugs. Some of these do not act on the cholinergic system, however. **Oxiracetam** and piracetam seem to enhance glutamate release (see below), and potentiate the activation of glutamate receptors of AMPA type; **xanthines** (Chapter 11) block the inhibitory modulator adenosine; and **denbufylline** inhibits phosphodiesterases. The effects of all these agents are small and inconsistent, both in normal people and Alzheimer's patients.

Other agents in the early stages of development include excitatory amino acid antagonists which may slow the rate of cell death; inverse agonists at benzodiazepine receptors which should oppose the effects of GABA and increase cholinergic neuron activity; and nerve growth factor, a peptide which seems to be essential for cholinergic neurons in the CNS to survive.

Attention is also being directed at preventing the formation of an insoluble protein, $\beta$-amyloid, which is deposited in the brains of Alzheimer's patients and is thought to disrupt neuronal function. The $\beta$-amyloid precursor protein is a normal constituent of cell membranes, consisting of a single transmembrane molecule of unknown function. In Alzheimer's disease this protein is split abnormally to yield the $\beta$-amyloid fragments which cannot be further metabolized and which therefore accumulates to an extent which ultimately kills the neurons.

## Noradrenaline/norepinephrine (NA/NE)

The synthesis and metabolism of NA/NE (see footnote page 24) proceeds as in the sympathetic nerve terminals (Figure 3.6) and neurons in the CNS can be localized either by antibodies to tyrosine hydroxylase or dopamine-$\beta$-hydroxylase, or by the formation of fluorescent derivatives after treating brain sections with formaldehyde. The major projection revealed originates in the locus coeruleus (LC, Figure 4.3) and ascends through the medial forebrain bundle to synapse throughout most regions of the cortex, with some branches also to the thalamus, hippocampus and cerebellum. The locus coeruleus is also known as the A6 region. A collection of smaller nuclei, A1, A5 and A7 have axons which join the forebrain projection, and an A2 group sends axons to influence the cardiac centres of the hindbrain.

### Receptors for NA/NE

Receptors for NA/NE are similar to the $\alpha$- and $\beta$-receptors found peripherally. Activation usually induces hyperpolarization, but with an accompanying increase of membrane resistance. There is also an inhibition of the calcium-activated potassium channel which causes the afterhyperpolarization following an action potential. The net effect is to reduce the spontaneous firing of neurons, but to enhance the responses to excitatory transmitters, increasing what is known as the neuronal signal–to–noise ratio.

Presynaptic $\alpha$2-receptors exist in the CNS, as in the periphery, usually on the terminals of noradrenergic and other neurons where they inhibit release of the transmitter. In addition, $\alpha$2-receptors occur on the cell bodies and dendrites of noradrenergic neurons in the locus coeruleus. When activated, for example by clonidine, these sites increase potassium conductance and thus suppress the firing of the cells. These **somatodendritic** receptors probably mediate the effects of several classes of drugs on the CNS, such as the centrally acting antihypertensives (clonidine, $\alpha$-methyldopa).

Although catecholaminergic neurons can be destroyed by injections of 6-hydroxydopamine, the behavioural role of central noradrenergic neurons is still unclear. They seem to be involved in complex activities requiring selective attention, and in the control of mood and motivation.

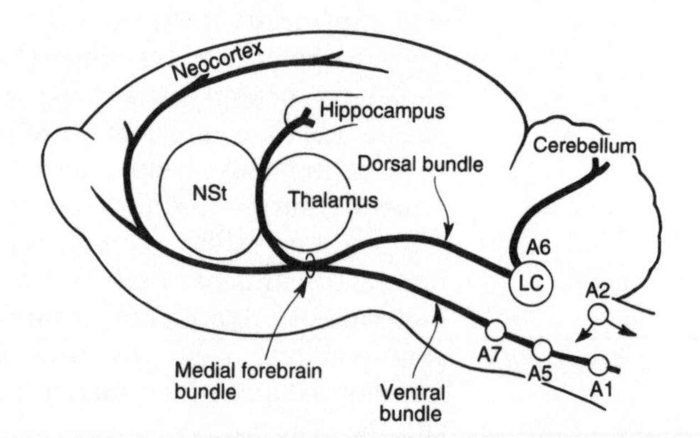


**Fig. 4.3** The major noradrenergic pathways in the CNS.LC, locus coeruleus.

## Dopamine

Another catecholamine, dopamine is synthesized from tyrosine (see Figure 3.6) but dopaminergic neurons lack the enzyme dopamine $\beta$-hydroxylase to convert it further into NA/NE. Dopamine itself is therefore transported into synaptic vesicles from where it can be released as a transmitter. After release, dopamine is inactivated primarily by reuptake (Uptake-1) which can be inhibited by drugs such as desipramine (Chapter 5) and nomifensine. Metabolism is similar to that of NA/NE, involving MAO and COMT, although dopamine is metabolized mainly by MAO-B (Chapter 3).

There are three major pathways in the CNS releasing dopamine as their neurotransmitter. The first arises from the substantia nigra (SN, Figure 4.4), also known as the A9 region, and projects to the (neo)striatum (NSt). It is this **nigrostriatal** pathway which is destroyed in Parkinson's disease (Chapter 8): the striatum is a major subcortical area for the control of voluntary and postural movements.

The second pathway ascends from the ventral tegmentum (VT, A10 area) to synapse in areas of the **limbic** system—the nucleus accumbens (NAcc), olfactory tubercle (OT) and frontal cortex (FC). This **mesolimbic** pathway is involved in mood and emotional responses and is disturbed in some affective and psychotic disorders.

The third dopaminergic pathway, (the tuberoinfundibular tract) travels from the hypothalamic A12 region to innervate the pituitary gland and control the release of prolactin (dopamine inhibits release).

### Receptors to dopamine

The two types of dopamine receptors studied most are D1 and D2, although other variants have been described. Their essential features are summarized in Table 4.1. Most of the effects of dopamine in the CNS are mediated by D2 receptors, and many of the drugs discussed in later chapters probably act here; it is likely that the D1 receptors have a subtler role to modulate D2 receptor function. The D3 and D4 receptors, which are localized to different regions of the mesolimbic system, may be important in psychiatric disorders (see Chapter 6). Most attention has been focussed on clozapine, which is one of the

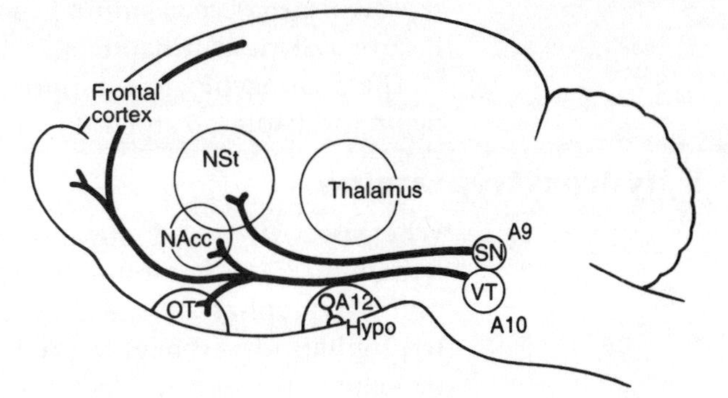


**Fig. 4.4** The major dopaminergic pathways in the CNS. SN, substantia nigra; VT, ventral tegmentum; OT, olfactory tubercle; NSt, neostriatum; NAcc, nucleus accumbens; Hypo, hypothalamus.

**Table 4.1** Dopamine receptors

| Receptor | G-protein | Transduction system | Sample location | Effects | Agonist | Antagonist |
|---|---|---|---|---|---|---|
| D1 | $G_s$ | Stimulation of adenylate cyclase | Postsynaptic in striatum | Hyperpolarization | SKF38393 | SCH23390 |
| | $G_q$ | Activation of PLC | | | | |
| D2 | $G_i/G_o$ | Inhibition of adenylate cyclase | Presynaptic (autoreceptors) and postsynaptic in striatum and limbic areas | Increase $gK^+$<br>Decrease $gCa^{++}$ | Quinpirole<br>Bromocriptine | Spiperone<br>(-) sulpiride<br>Haloperidol |
| D3 | $G_i/G_o$ | Inhibition of adenylate cyclase | Limbic system | ? | Quinpirole<br>Bromocriptine | Spiperone |
| D4 | $G_i/G_o$ | Inhibition of adenylate cyclase | Frontal cortex, mid-brain, amygdala | ? | – | Clozapine<br>Spiperone |
| D5 | $G_s$ | Stimulation of adenylate cyclase | Hypothalamus, hippocampus | ? | SKF38393 | SCH23390 |

most potent and effective antipsychotic drugs available and which shows a higher affinity for D4 receptors.

All the dopamine receptors belong to the G-protein coupled superfamily with seven transmembrane-spanning sequences. There is at least a 50% homology between the intramembrane regions of the various receptors.

In studying the functions of dopamine containing neurons, use is made of a toxic compound, 6-hydroxydopamine which is taken up into the neurons and causes their death. The behaviour of animals lacking dopamine neurons can then be compared with normal animals.

In rodents, stimulation of striatal dopamine receptors unilaterally causes the animals to walk around in circles; this rotation behaviour is a useful test of striatal dopamine function. Activation of dopamine receptors also causes repeated, stereotyped sniffing and licking behaviours which resemble those of tardive dyskinesia (Chapter 6).

The pharmacological importance of dopamine will be explored in greater depth in Chapters 6 and 8.

## 5-Hydroxytryptamine

Whereas NA/NE and dopamine are catechol-derived amines, 5-hydroxytryptamine (5HT; serotonin) is an indoleamine. It is synthesized from the amino acid L-tryptophan by the enzymes tryptophan hydroxylase and 5-hydroxytryptophan decarboxylase (Figure 4.5) and is metabolized mainly by monoamine oxidase A. Tryptophan hydroxylase is the rate-limiting enzyme and

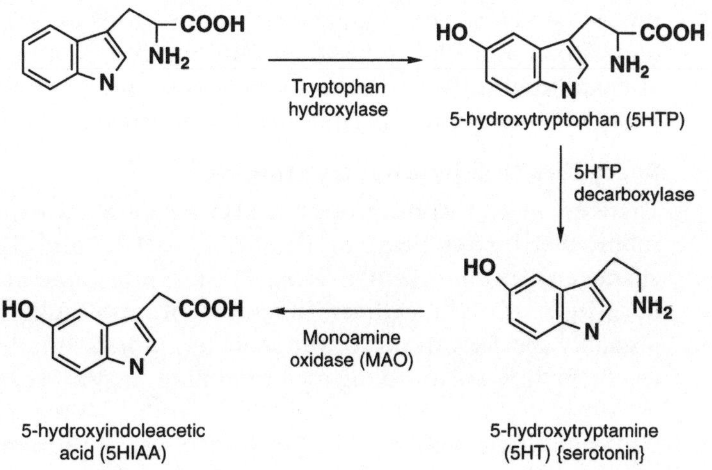

COOH
$NH_2$
N
Tryptophan hydroxylase
HO
COOH
$NH_2$
N
5-hydroxytryptophan (5HTP)
5HTP decarboxylase
HO
$NH_2$
N
HO
COOH
N
Monoamine oxidase (MAO)
5-hydroxyindoleacetic acid (5HIAA)
5-hydroxytryptamine (5HT) {serotonin}

**Fig. 4.5** Synthesis and metabolism of 5-hydroxytyptamine (5HT or serotonin).

can be inhibited by *p*-chlorophenylalanine, which thus depletes neurons of 5HT and has been used to study the functional role of 5HT neurons. Reserpine affects these terminals as well as catecholamine synapses, preventing the storage of 5HT within synaptic vesicles, and thus causing depletion of 5HT stores. Similarly, amphetamine (Chapter 3) triggers the release of 5HT, as well as catecholamines. Once released 5HT is primarily removed from the extracellular space by uptake into the nerve terminal, a process which can be inhibited by drugs such as **fluoxetine** (Chapter 5). The amine can then be recycled into synaptic vesicles, or metabolised by MAO-A (Figure 4.5).

The hydroxylated compound 5, 7-dihydroxytryptamine is taken up into 5HT neurons but subsequently causes their death. The mechanism is unclear but may involve free radicals. As with 6-hydroxydopamine, this toxin is useful in determining the biological roles of 5HT containing neurons.

The main sites of origin of 5HT neuronal pathways are the dorsal (B7) and medial (B8) raphe nuclei (RN, Figure 4.6) which project axons through the medial forebrain bundle to most brain regions, including the cortex and

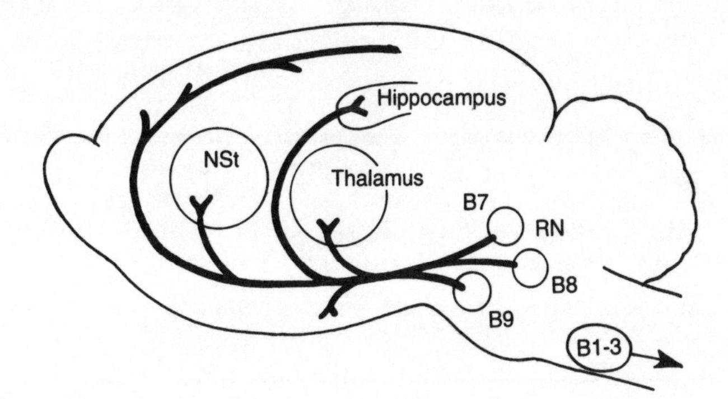


**Fig. 4.6** The major serotoninergic pathways in the CNS. RN, raphe nuclei; NSt neostriatum.

hippocampus. The overall behavioural functions of 5HT neurons are not fully understood, but they seem to mediate inhibition of behavioural responses—after destroying the neurons animals respond more eagerly and rapidly to environmental stimuli, even if they are punished as a result!

### Receptors to 5-hydroxytryptamine

There are at least three groups of 5HT receptors, the first of which has been subdivided into at least $5HT_{1A}$, $5HT_{1B}$, $5HT_{1C}$ and $5HT_{1D}$ subtypes. Some characteristics are shown in Table 4.2. The $5HT_{1B}$ and $5HT_{1D}$ subtypes seem to have such similar locations, functions and molecular biology that they are probably species variants of the same receptor. Similarly the $5HT_{1C}$ and $5HT_2$ receptors show such striking molecular homology and properties that they may be considered variants of a single population. All the receptors possess seven transmembrane regions and are linked via G-proteins to their respective transduction systems (Chapter 1, and Table 4.2).

**Table 4.2** 5-hydroxytryptamine receptors

| Receptor | Neuronal location and function | CNS location | Behavioural involvement | G-protein | Transduction system | Agonists | Antagonists |
|---|---|---|---|---|---|---|---|
| $5HT_{1A}$ | Presynaptic (inhibitory autoreceptors); postsynaptic | Hippocampus; raphe nuclei | Anxiety, Depression, Appetite, Sexual | $G_i/G_o$ | Inhibition of adenylate cyclase; open $K^+$ channels | 8-hydroxy-DPAT Ipsapirone | Propranolol |
| $5HT_{1B}$ $5HT_{1D}$ | Presynaptic: -1B in rodents -1D other species, inhibition of transmitter release; vasoconstriction | Basal ganglia (subs. nigra, pallidum) | Anxiety, Appetite | $G_i/G_o$ | inhibition of adenylate cyclase | Sumatriptan | Cyanopindolol |
| $5HT_{1C}$ | Postsynaptic | Striatum, limbic areas, choroid plexus | Appetite | $G_q$ or $G_i/G_o$ | Activation of PLC | α-methyl-5HT | Propranolol Ketanserin Mesulergine |
| $5HT_2$ | Postsynaptic (depolarization) | Cerebral cortex | Nociception, Cognitive function Hallucinogenesis | $G_q$ or $G_i/G_o$ | Activation of PLC; Closure of $K^+$ channels | α-methyl-5HT, LSD | Ketanserin Ritanserin |
| $5HT_3$ | Postsynaptic (depolarization) | Cortex, limbic areas, hindbrain (vagal afferent) | Anxiety, memory, emesis cognitive function | – | Ligand-gated ion channel for cations | 2-methyl-5HT | Ondansetron Granisetron Zacopride |
| $5HT_4$ | Postsynaptic (depolarization) | Hippocampus, Cerebral cortex | ? | $G_s$ | Stimulation of adenylate cyclase; closure of $K^+$ channels | 2-methyl-5HT | Tropisetron |

The $5HT_{1A}$ receptors are widely distributed throughout the CNS and some of the drugs which act on them have striking behavioural effects. Agonists, such as **buspirone**, for example, are good anxiolytics. These receptors also occur in the hippocampus, where they may modulate learning processes, and are associated with hypothalamic autonomic centres controlling body temperature and sexual activity. $5HT_{1A}$ receptors occur on the cell bodies and dendrites of raphe neurons; these somatodendritic receptors depress the firing of the raphe cells and thus inhibit activity in most of the 5HT pathways.

Migraine is thought to be due to a dilatation of blood vessels in the head, possibly associated with, or even caused by, a degree of local inflammation. The $5HT_{1D}$ receptor occurs in association with cerebral blood vessels and their activation can cause contraction and reduce the release of local inflammatory mediators. **Sumatriptan** is a selective agonist at these sites and as a result is able to reduce rapidly the nausea and severe headaches of migraine.

$5HT_2$ receptors seem to be concerned with general arousal and cognitive functions: antagonists diminish fatigue and have an antidepressant effect in some depressed patients and schizophrenic subjects. The hallucinogenic effects of drugs such as LSD and mescaline (Chapter 11) appear to be mediated by $5HT_2$ receptors. The receptors can be blocked selectively by agents such as **ritanserin** (Figure 4.7).

$5HT_3$ receptors are widely distributed in the brain, and have many potential functions. Antagonists at these sites are markedly anxiolytic in animal tests,

**Table 4.3** Properties of glutamate receptors

| Receptor | Subunit components | Trans-membrane regions | G-protein | Transduction system |
|---|---|---|---|---|
| NMDA | NMDAR1 | 4 | – | Ligand-gated |
| | NMDAR2A | 4 | | ion channel: |
| | NMDAR2B | 4 | | $Na^+$, $Ca^{++}$ |
| | NMDAR2C | 4 | | |
| | NMDAR2D | 4 | | |
| AMPA | GluR1 | 4 | – | Ligand-gated |
| | GluR2 | 4 | | ion channel: |
| | GluR3 | 4 | | $Na^+$, $K^+$, ($Ca^{++}$) |
| | GluR4 | 4 | | |
| Kainate | GluR5 | 4 | – | Ligand-gated |
| | GluR6 | 4 | | ion channel: |
| | GluR7 | 4 | | $Na^+$, $Ca^{++}$ |
| | KA1, KA2 | 4 | | |
| Metabotropic | mGluR1 | 7 | $G_q$ or $G_i/G_o$ | Activates PLC |
| | mGluR2 | 7 | $G_i/G_o$ | Inhibit adenylate |
| | mGluR3 | 7 | $G_i/G_o$ | cyclase |
| | mGluR4 | 7 | $G_i/G_o$ | |
| | mGluR5 | 7 | $G_q$ or $G_i/G_o$ | Activates PLC |
| | mGluR6 | 7 | $G_i/G_o$ | Inhibit adenylate cyclase |

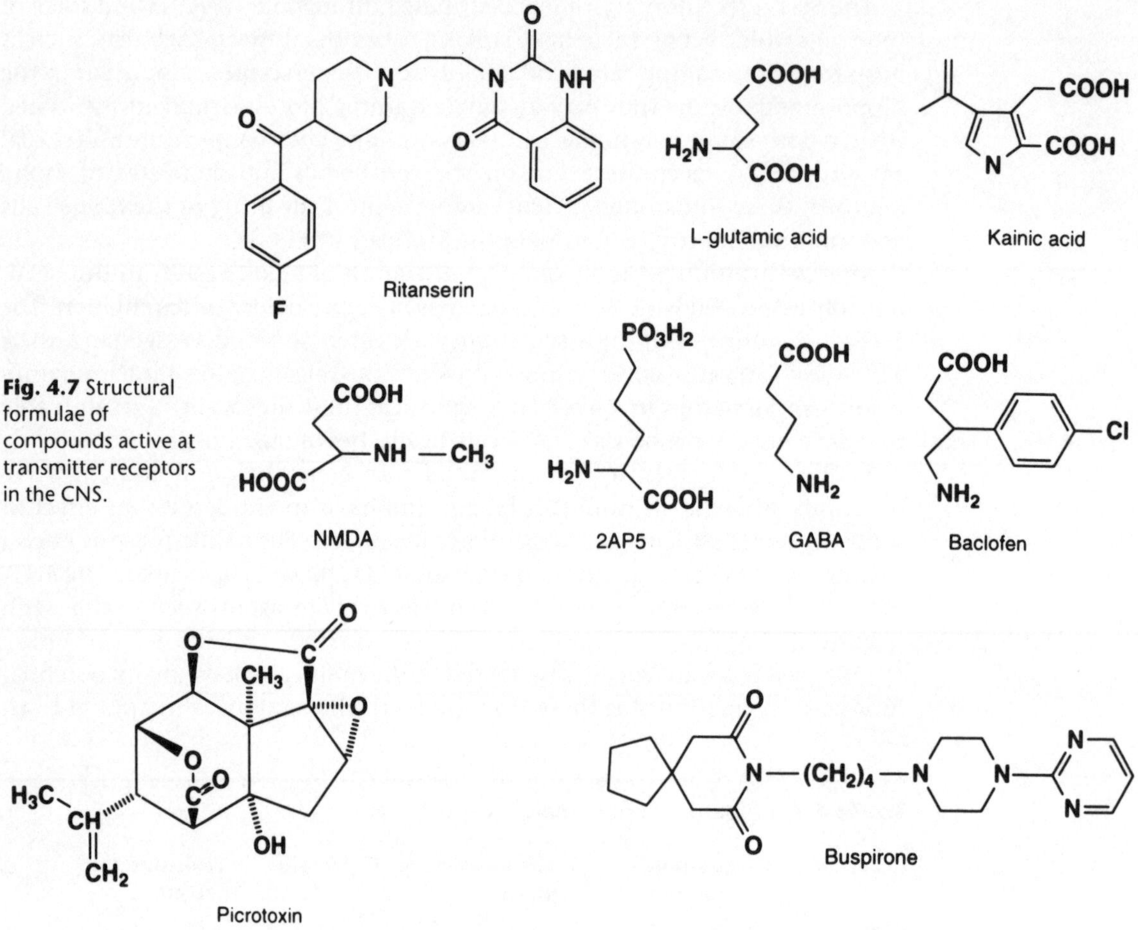

Ritanserin

L-glutamic acid

Kainic acid

NMDA

2AP5

GABA

Baclofen

Picrotoxin

Buspirone

Arg-Pro-Lys-Pro-Gln-Gln-Phe-Phe-Gly-Leu-Met-$NH_2$
Substance P

**Fig. 4.7** Structural formulae of compounds active at transmitter receptors in the CNS.

probably due to blockade in limbic areas such as the amygdala. Antagonists also improve cognitive performance ('intelligent' behaviour) in rodents or primates, when faced with complex learning or discrimination tasks. For these reasons $5HT_3$ antagonists are being actively developed as anxiolytic and nootropic (cognition-enhancing) drugs respectively.

Some $5HT_3$ receptors are also located on and around the terminals of vagal afferent axons in the hindbrain (nucleus tractus solitarius). Afferent vagal information is normally involved in triggering vomiting, and $5HT_3$ antagonists suppress vomiting, even when induced by powerful emetic stimulants such as radiation therapy (for cancer) or the anti-cancer drug cisplatin.

A recently described $5HT_4$ receptor has been identified on several peripheral tissues as well as in the hippocampus and frontal cerebral cortex. This site seems to promote depolarization of neurons and contraction of intestinal and cardiac muscle.

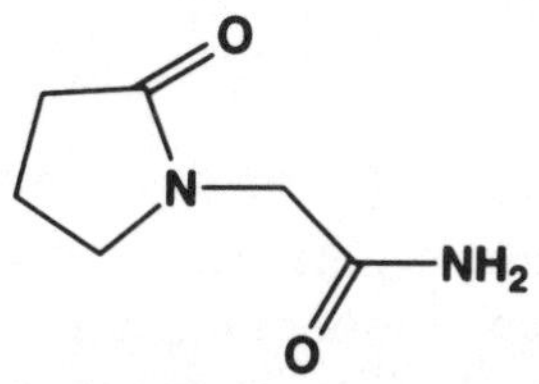

Piracetam

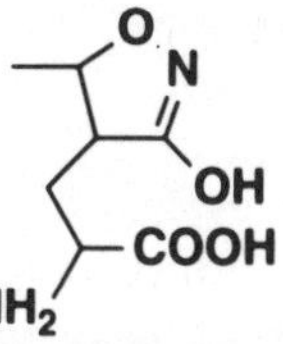

AMPA

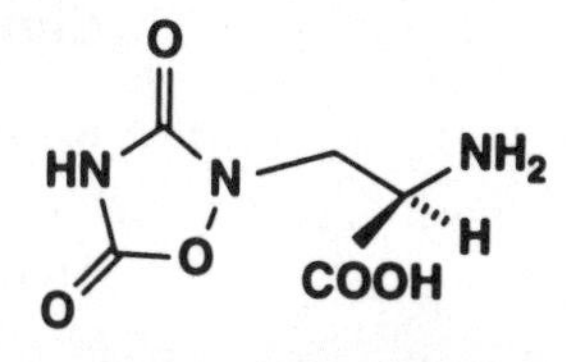

Quisqualic acid

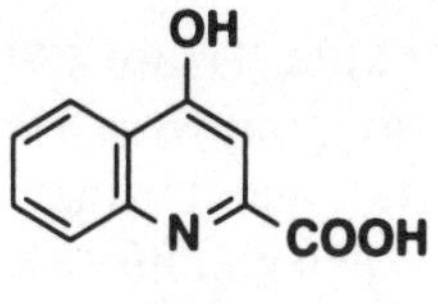

Kynurenic acid

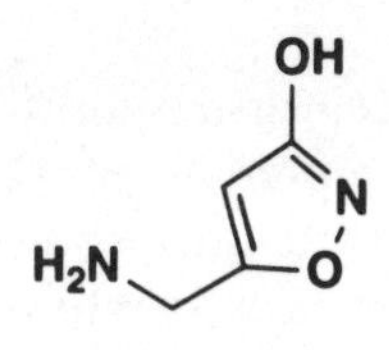

Muscimol

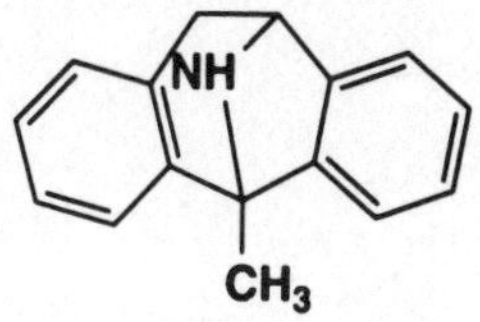

Dizocilpine
(MK-801)

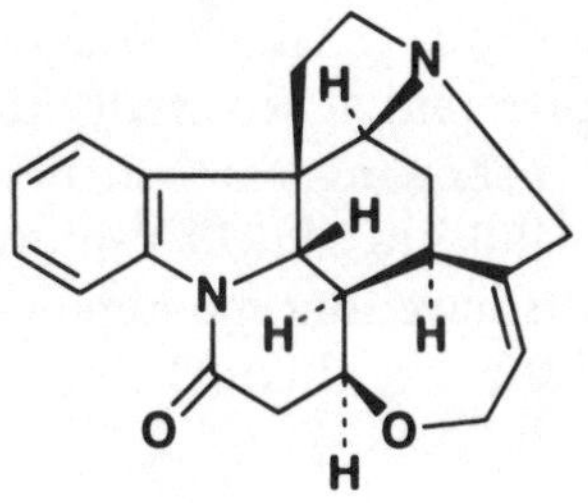

Strychnine

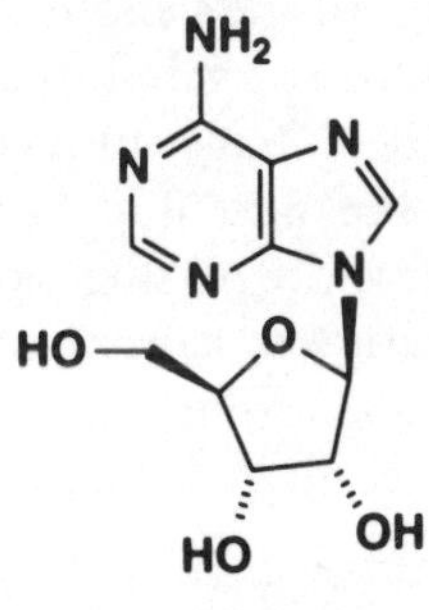

Adenosine

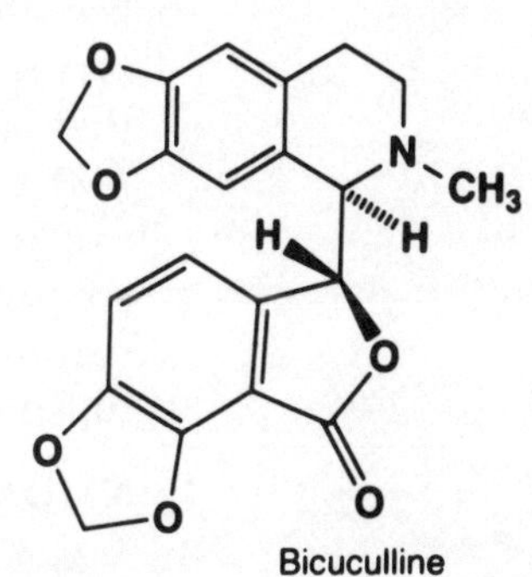

Bicuculline

## Glutamic acid

It is believed that simple amino acid transmitters such as glutamate and GABA are involved in the vast majority of synapses in the CNS. Glutamate (Figure 4.7) is synthesized either *de novo* from glucose, or from glutamine which is taken up into the nerve terminal after being formed in glial cells from previously released glutamate (the glutamine cycle). Glutamate itself can also be taken back up into the synaptic terminals by a high affinity uptake process, equivalent to the Uptake-1 systems of aminergic neurons.

Glutamatergic neurons are widely distributed throughout the CNS and include both short interneurons and long projection pathways—the corticofugal neurons from the motor cerebral cortex to the lower spinal cord release glutamate and are among the longest neurons in the body. Once released, glutamate (the L-isomer) causes depolarization and thus excitation of neurons, but it does so by acting on a variety of receptors, which are best described separately.

## Glutamate receptors

### Kainate receptor

One receptor responds best to the glutamate analogue kainic acid (Figure 4.7). An increase of cation conductance is produced which causes depolarization. The effect is quite long-lasting, however, and a significant amount of calcium may enter the cells and potentially cause damage (see later). The kainate receptors can be blocked by compounds such as 6,7-dinitroquinoxaline-2,3-dione (DNQX).

### AMPA receptor

A separate group of receptors respond to another analogue, AMPA (Figure 4.7) which also raises cation permeability and causes depolarization, but with less effect on calcium, and for a much shorter duration. Both the AMPA and kainate receptors seem to play critical roles in synaptic transmission. When glutamate is released as a transmitter it usually produces a rapid, short-latency depolarization which is mediated by these receptors.

The pharmacological properties of AMPA and kainate receptors overlap because the structures of the various subunits of which they are composed are very similar (Table 4.3). The subunits are referred to as GluR1 to GluR7. Four of them (GluR1 to GluR4) make up receptors with a preferential sensitivity to AMPA, and exist in 'flip' and 'flop' variants, the former showing less tendency to desensitize and therefore passing more current. The GluR5 to GluR7 receptors are particularly sensitive to kainate. All these subunits have four membrane-spanning sections, consistent with membership of the ion channel linked superfamily.

### NMDA receptor

*N*-Methyl-D-aspartate (NMDA) is the preferred agonist at a fourth group of receptors. The receptor belongs to the ion-channel linked superfamily, the associated channel passing sodium and calcium ions. Accordingly, the receptor components each have four transmembrane-spanning sequences, and so far five distinct subunits have been identified. These are the NMDAR1 and NMDAR2A to D subunits, which are able to form a number of functional homomeric (consisting of several molecules of the same subunits) or heteromeric (made up of different subunits) receptors with rather special features.

As illustrated in Figure 4.8, these are complex receptors with several attachment sites for agents which are able to modulate receptor activity. Besides the binding site for NMDA (or, normally, glutamate) there are sites for glycine and polyamines which enhance, or may be necessary for, receptor activity. The receptor is coupled to an ionic channel which can pass sodium and calcium ions, resulting in depolarization, but which is partially blocked by magnesium ions. As neurons are depolarized by other means (acetylcholine, or activation of AMPA receptors, for example) the block by magnesium is reduced—it is a **voltage-dependent** blockade.

Under normal circumstances, then, glutamate probably excites cells mainly by the kainate and AMPA receptors. If depolarization is large, or prolonged, the

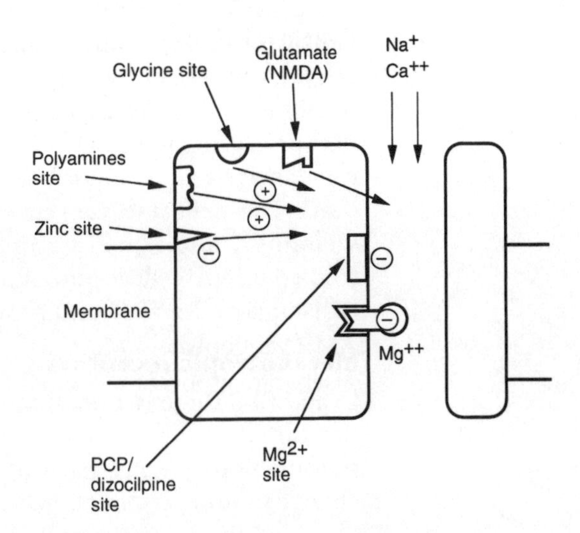


**Fig. 4.8** A diagrammatic representation of the NMDA receptor for glutamate. Receptor activation is facilitated by a strychnine-insensitive glycine receptor and a polyamine site. The receptor can be blocked by zinc or by blockade of the channel by magnesium ions, phencyclidine (PCP) or dizocilpine.

magnesium channel blockade is reduced and NMDA receptors play a progressively greater part in synaptic transmission. As a result, NMDA receptors are very important in CNS function.

(**a**) convulsions (Chapter 8) involve excessive firing of neurons and will recruit NMDA receptors, helping to maintain and prolong the seizures. NMDA antagonists may be useful antiepileptic drugs.

(**b**) learning is thought to involve long-term changes of neuronal excitability following rapidly repeated or coincident stimuli. NMDA receptors could mediate such a phenomenon, and NMDA antagonists do interfere with some forms of memory.

(**c**) the prolonged influx of calcium ions through NMDA channels can cause cell damage, and it is known that glutamate receptors, including NMDA receptors are overactivated during cerebral ischaemia or haemorrhage (strokes), mechanical brain injury or hypoglycaemia. NMDA receptors may thus be responsible for much of the brain damage produced by these insults and antagonists are likely to be important inhibitors of brain damage, neuroprotectants, in the next century. Compounds which block NMDA receptors competitively at the receptor site such as 2-amino-5-phosphonopentanoic acid (2AP5, Figure 4.7) or which block the associate ion channels (e.g. dizocilpine, [MK 801]; Figure 4.7) are being used as lead compounds in developing drugs for this purpose. Antagonists acting at the glycine modulatory site, such as kynurenic acid, also look promising.

## Free radicals

In many cases there is evidence to suggest that the elevation of intracellular calcium produced by glutamate receptor activation (especially kainate and NMDA receptors) can cause the formation of free radicals such as the hydroxyl radical ($OH^{\bullet}$). Free radicals include atoms which lack one electron in the outer orbital. Consequently they are highly unstable and will steal an electron from other molecules such as membrane lipids, proteins or nucleic acids. This in turn, of course, generates a new free radical so that a chain reaction is initiated which can damage a large number of vital molecules and lead to severe cell damage or death. Free radical scavengers which neutralize these injurious particles, such as vitamins C and E and a number of synthetic analogues of them, are being studied intensively as potential inhibitors of cell damage following trauma or ischaemia of the brain and heart.

### Metabotropic receptors

In addition there is a population of metabotropic receptors, so called because the initial result of their activation is a stimulation of second messenger transduction systems, especially of phospholipase C (Figure 1.6) rather than a change of ionic conductance as in the case of the other, ionotropic receptors discussed above. These receptors possess seven transmembrane regions and are coupled to G-proteins (Table 4.3). However, the activation of these receptors does cause slow, delayed changes of ionic conductance which are probably the result of activating PLC. These changes include blocking calcium-dependent and voltage-dependent potassium currents and the M current.

### Gamma-aminobutyric acid

Gamma-aminobutyric acid (GABA) (Figure 4.7) is synthesized from glutamate by glutamate decarboxylase (GAD) and antibodies to this enzyme are often used to localize GABA containing neurons or synaptic terminals. GABA is the dominant inhibitory neurotransmitter in the CNS. After release from neurons it is taken up by a high-affinity uptake process which can be inhibited by nipecotic acid. GABA can then be recycled back into synaptic vesicles or metabolized by GABA-transaminase (GABA-T). Inhibitors of this enzyme (such as vigabatrin, Chapter 8) thus increase neuronal concentrations of GABA and facilitate inhibitory transmission.

GABA acts on at least two types of receptor, $GABA_A$ and $GABA_B$ (Table 4.4). $GABA_A$ receptors are made up of subunits, of which 14 varieties have been

**Table 4.4** GABA receptors

| Receptor | Location | Transduction system | Effects | Agonists | Antagonists |
|---|---|---|---|---|---|
| $GABA_A$ | CNS; mainly postsynaptic | Ligand-gated ion channel | Increased chloride conductance; neuronal inhibition | GABA muscimol | Bicuculline Picrotoxin (channel block) |
| $GABA_B$ | Presynaptic and postsynaptic | $G_i/G_o$ | Inhibition of adenylate cyclase; increase of $gK^+$; decrease of $gCa^{++}$ | GABA Baclofen | Phaclofen 2-hydroxy-saclofen |

discovered: $\alpha1$ to $\alpha6$, $\beta1$ to $\beta3$, $\gamma1$ to $\gamma3$, $\delta$ and $\rho$. Selections of these occur, providing a potentially large number of receptor combinations. Activation of $GABA_A$ receptors leads to an increase in chloride permeability and thus hyperpolarization. Antagonists at $GABA_A$ receptors, such as bicuculline and picrotoxin, increase excitability in the CNS and may cause convulsions.

$GABA_B$ receptors usually increase potassium conductance, again causing hyperpolarization of neurons. This effect is mediated by G-proteins (Table 4.4)

A number of important drugs, such as benzodiazepines and barbiturates act by potentiating GABA-mediated inhibition and are discussed in more detail later (see Chapter 7). Benzodiazepine effects result from their binding to a gamma subunit, whereas GABA itself binds to the $\alpha$-subunits.

## Glycine

Glycine (the simplest amino acid, $NH_2CH_2COOH$) is an inhibitory transmitter in the hindbrain and spinal cord where its ligand-gated ion channel receptors are blocked by the convulsant alkaloid **strychnine** (Figure 4.7). The receptors are pentameric, made from $\alpha$ and $\beta$ subunits: the $\alpha$ subunits binds glycine, while the $\beta$ subunit determines channel conductance. Each subunit has four transmembrane regions.

Glycine is the transmitter released by the recurrent inhibitory Renshaw cells onto ventral horn motoneurons (Figure 4.2) where it causes hyperpolarization and prevents excessive firing of the motoneurons. By blocking this inhibitory feedback, strychnine can cause convulsions which may lead to death from muscular exhaustion and respiratory failure.

Glycine also binds to a modulatory site on the glutamate NMDA receptor (Figure 4.8) which facilitates activation of the receptor/channel complex. This site is ***not*** blocked by strychnine, but is blocked by the tryptophan metabolite, kynurenic acid (Figure 4.7).

## Peptides

A number of peptides exist in synaptic terminals in the CNS and have potent effects on neuronal firing. They include substance P, cholecystokinin, neurotensin, neuropeptide Y and somatostatin, as well as the releasing factors thyrotrophin and corticotrophin releasing hormones and the opioid peptides discussed in Chapter 9. Most of these peptides co-exist with the 'classical' transmitters described above and are released from the same neurons (co-transmission). They are often released only with more intense neuronal activity and many have prolonged actions. Several of the following have been introduced in Chapter 3.

### Substance P

Substance P is one of the tachykinin family of peptides (page 43). In the CNS, substance P is one of the most likely candidates as the transmitter of some small diameter C-fibre primary afferent sensory neurons entering the dorsal horn of the spinal cord. The peptide is present in the dorsal horn, but concentrations decrease after separating the dorsal root ganglia from the cord. Neuronal responses to noxious afferent stimulation of mechanical or chemical receptors in the skin can be partially blocked by antagonists at NK2 receptors, although responses to noxious thermal stimuli are unaffected. Antagonists at NK2 receptors are being developed as potential non-opioid (and therefore perhaps non-addicting) analgesics.

The compound **capsaicin** (from peppers) produces depolarization of substance P-containing afferents (hence the painful sensations of eating peppers). Repeated use of capsaicin, however, can destroy nociceptive afferents. An antagonist at capsaicin receptors, **capsazepine**, is being studied as a potential analgesic.

In the brain, substance P appears to be a transmitter in neuronal pathways from the caudate nucleus to the substantia nigra, from raphe nuclei to the cord, and in the amygdala. The first of these is of particular interest since modulation of substance P activity may be useful in treating Parkinson's disease (Chapter 8).

## Cholecystokinin

In the CNS, cholecystokinin (CCK) exists mainly as the sulfated octapeptide CCK-8S. It acts upon two varieties of receptor, CCK-A and CCK-B. The former is found mainly on peripheral tissues (pancreas, gall-bladder, gastrointestinal muscle) whereas CCK-B sites are the predominant variety in the CNS , where they are coupled via a Gq protein to the activation of phospholipase C.

CCK produces a powerful depolarization of neurons in the brain, and is involved in several important behaviours. Pathways within the CNS, for example, seem to be involved in satiety, and thus regulate the intake of food. Injections of CCK directly into the brain cause antinociception in animals, with a potency greater than morphine. There is evidence also that antagonists at CCK-B receptors can potentiate opiate antinociception but suppress the development of tolerance. CCK receptor ligands may thus find use as anti-appetite drugs or analgesic agents.

Finally, some anxiolytic benzodiazepines (Chapter 7) block CCK receptors, and injections of CCK agonists into humans induces feelings of intense anxiety and panic. Some drugs, such as CI 998, which is a selective antagonist at CCK-B receptors, are therefore being developed as novel anxiolytic drugs.

## Somatostatin

In the CNS receptors for somatostatin (SST) (page 44) are coupled via Gi-proteins to the inhibition of adenylate cyclase. They can also increase potassium conductance, again via a G-protein, to produce hyperpolarization and can reduce calcium permeability leading to inhibition of release of some transmitters such as NA/NE and GABA. SST is often co-localized in the same neurons as NA/NE or GABA.

There are several long projection pathways containing SST in the CNS, between limbic regions, the neocortex, locus coeruleus and substantia nigra, and it also exists in primary afferent sensory neurons. In the latter case, stimulation by noxious heat but not mechanical or chemical stimuli causes SST release, and neuronal responses to noxious heat are blocked by SST antagonists. SST also seems to be involved in the regulation of sleep and locomotor activity. SST levels are increased as a result of repeated seizures in animals and humans, and antagonists or antibodies to SST are anticonvulsant. Finally, SST concentration is greatly reduced in the cerebral cortex of Alzheimer patients, a finding which may have implications for the treatment of this disorder.

### Angiotensin

Angiotensin is best known for its peripheral effects on vascular tone and aldosterone secretion, but neurons containing elements of the angiotensin system are found in regions of the CNS around the cerebral ventricles (the circumventricular organs), areas which also contain angiotensin receptors. These areas lack a blood–brain barrier, so that the receptors may be affected by angiotensin released locally or penetrating from the blood stream. Receptors are of two types, AT1 and AT2. AT1 sites are primarily sensitive to angiotensin II, and are subdivided into $AT1_A$ receptors which inhibit adenylate cyclase and $AT1_B$ receptors which activate phospholipase C. AT2 receptors inhibit guanylate cyclase. All these receptors are coupled to the transduction systems by G-proteins.

The importance of the angiotensin receptors seems to lie in their control of water intake. Stimulation of the receptors will initiate drinking behaviour very rapidly, a phenomenon consistent with the overall body function of angiotensin to regulate blood volume and osmolarity.

## Purines

The purine nucleoside **adenosine** is found throughout the nervous system and is released as a result of neuronal depolarization, but not necessarily from vesicles, as a neurotransmitter. In fact adenosine is probably the clearest example of a neuromodulator although it does have inhibitory effects of its own on neuronal activity, mainly the result of increasing potassium conductances. In addition, it can modulate receptor sensitivity to other transmitters, notably acetylcholine NA/NE and dopamine. It also depresses transmitter release, especially of excitatory agents such as glutamate and acetylocholine.

These various effects are produced by three receptor subtypes (Table 3.4). The A1 receptors are G-protein coupled to inhibit adenylate cyclase, but they are also responsible for the increases of potassium currents and the suppression of transmitter release. Several selective agonists are available for these sites, including $N^6$-cyclopentyladenosine, which possess cyclic substituents on the nitrogen atom at position 6. The A2 receptors are G-protein linked to the stimulation of adenylate cyclase, and they also increase the release of some transmitters. Selective agonists include $N^6$-[2-(3,5-dimethoxyphenyl)-2-(2-methylphenyl)-ethyl]adenosine (DPMA). The stimulant effects of xanthines such as caffeine (Chapter 11) are due to blocking the effects of adenosine in the CNS. Some xanthines are selective antagonists at A1 or A2 receptors. The A3 receptors for adenosine have not yet been studied in detail.

Selective agonists at A1 receptors are anticonvulsant, antinociceptive and protect against brain damage produced by excitatory amino acids or ischaemia. Antagonists may be valuable as cognition enhancers in the elderly, or in the treatment of patients with Alzheimer's disease.

# 5 Affective disorders: antidepressant drugs

## Introduction

The noun affect means mood or feelings. Affective disorders are disturbances of the psychiatric state of patients characterized by changes in mood or emotional state and depression is a common example.

Most people experience a brief period of depression at some time in their lives, which can often be directly attributed to a particular circumstance such as a bereavement, redundancy or a failed examination. This is normal. The pathological state of major, endogenous or chronic depression either has no obvious cause, or is far more profound and long-lasting than is appropriate for a particular triggering event. Depressed patients experience intense sadness, a sense of hopelessness and personal inadequacy, reflected in a withdrawal from society and personal relationships, and often accompanied by general apathy, slow, laboured movements and a serious loss of appetite, sleep, libido and ability to concentrate. In extreme cases endogenous depression can result in suicide.

### Causes of depression

Some of the first clues to the neurochemical cause of depression came earlier this century from the occurrence of severe depression in patients being treated with reserpine (Figure 3.8), an active alkaloid extracted from the plant *Rauwolfia serpentina*, for hypertension. Reserpine prevents the storage of amines, including the catecholamines dopamine, AD/E and NA/NE and the indoleamine (Chapters 3 and 4) in synaptic vesicles, leading to a transient increase in their release, followed by a prolonged period of amine depletion. (Its anti-hypertensive effect is largely due to the depletion of NA/NE from synaptic nerve terminals.) As reserpine can cross the blood–brain barrier this depletion also occurs in the CNS.

In parallel with the realization that reserpine caused depression came the discovery that some patients being treated with the anti-tuberculosis drug **iproniazid** exhibited an elevation in their mood—a degree of euphoria. Iproniazid was soon found to have the opposite neurochemical effect to reserpine—it raised amine concentrations in neurons by inhibiting the main enzyme responsible for amine metabolism, monoamine oxidase (MAO). Thus was born the Monoamine Hypothesis of depression: a deficiency of monoamines in the CNS causes depression and an increase of amines relieves depression. It is of course difficult to measure the amine levels in the brain of living humans, but measurements of their metabolities, such as 3-methoxy-4-hydroxyphenylglycol (Chapter 3) have confirmed a significant lowering of concentration in the urine and CSF of depressed patients, and a return to normal levels on drug treatment and clinical recovery.

# Current drugs

The drugs currently available for treating endogenous depression fall into three general groups : (1) monoamine oxidase inhibitors; (2) Uptake-1 inhibitors; and (3) atypical drugs.

## Monoamine oxidase inhibitors

The first group is the monoamine oxidase (MAO) inhibitors such as iproniazid (Table 5.1; Figures 5.1A and 5.2) though these drugs are being used less frequently in the clinic because of their side effects. These compounds produce

**Table 5.1** Antidepressant drugs

| Drug types | Notes |
|---|---|
| **MAO inhibitors: non-selective** | |
| Iproniazid | Associated with clinical delay, |
| Pargyline | |
| Isocarboxazid | muscarinic blockade, hypotension, |
| Tranylcypromine | |
| Phenelzine | CNS stimulation, 'cheese reaction' |
| **MAO inhibitors: selective** | |
| Clorgyline | MAO-A inhibitor |
| **Amine uptake inhibitors** | |
| Imipramine | Tricyclic antidepressants (TADs); |
| Desipramine | clinical delay, sedation, muscarinic |
| Amitriptyline | blockade, cardiac dysrhythmias. |
| Nortriptyline | |
| **Selective NA/NE uptake inhibitors** | |
| Maprotiline | Tetracyclic structure |
| Oxaprotiline | |
| **Selective 5HT uptake inhibitors** | |
| Zimelidine | |
| Citalopram | |
| Fluvoxamine | |
| Fluoxetine | |
| **Atypical antidepressants** | |
| Mianserin | Tetracyclic; $\alpha_2$-antagonist |
| Iprindole | |
| Bupropion | Facilitates dopamine release |
| Nomifensine | Inhibits dopamine and NA/NE uptake |

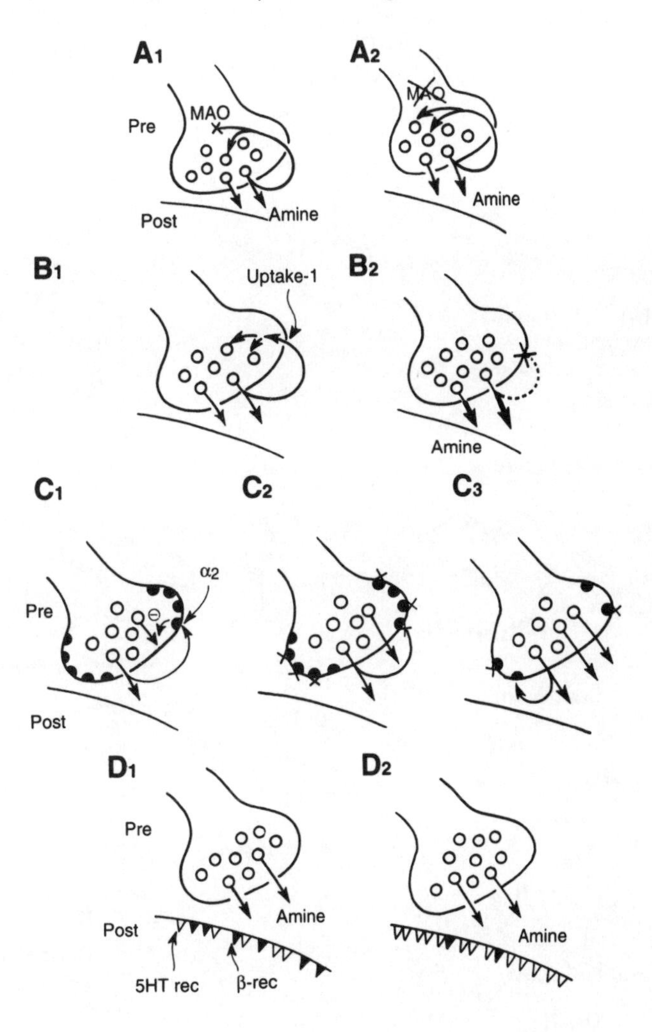


**Fig. 5.1** Mechanism of action of antidepressant drugs. (A1) Monoamine oxidase normally destroys some of the amines synthesized in, or taken up into nerve terminals. Inhibition of the enzyme increases the amount of amine which can be released onto postsynaptic receptors (A2). (B1) Uptake-1 is normally responsible for reducing the extracellular concentration of amines. (B2) Inhibition of uptake-1 enhances aminergic transmission. (C1) Stimulation of presynaptic $\alpha$-2 receptors normally suppresses excessive amine release. Blockade of these (C2) increases amine release and this may in turn further reduce receptor number (C3). (D1) Released monoamines normally cause activation of a variety of receptors (directly or indirectly), including $\alpha$-adrenoceptors and 5HT receptors. Many antidepressant drugs lead to a down-regulation of $\beta$-receptors and up-regulation of 5HT receptors, (D2).

an increase of amine concentration in the synaptic terminals. They probably do not increase transmitter release following action potentials, but may cause a 'leakage' of amine onto the postsynaptic receptors.

Most compounds available in this class inhibit both known forms of MAO—$MAO_A$ and $MAO_B$ and are therefore non-selective. $MAO_A$ is mainly responsible for metabolizing NA/NE and 5HT, whereas $MAO_B$ prefers to oxidize phenylethylamine and dopamine. The predominant form of MAO in the human brain is $MAO_B$ but selective $MAO_B$ inhibitors do not appear to be antidepressant. Selective $MAO_A$ inhibitors such as **clorgyline** (Figure 5.2) on the other hand are effective antidepressants, supporting the view that it is the NA/NE and 5HT neurotransmitter systems which are primarily involved in depression.

Although some MAO inhibitors such as **tranylcypromine** are reversible, others such as **phenelzine** and **isocarboxazid** (Figure 5.2) become covalently bound to the enzyme, being themselves destroyed. As a result, recovery from

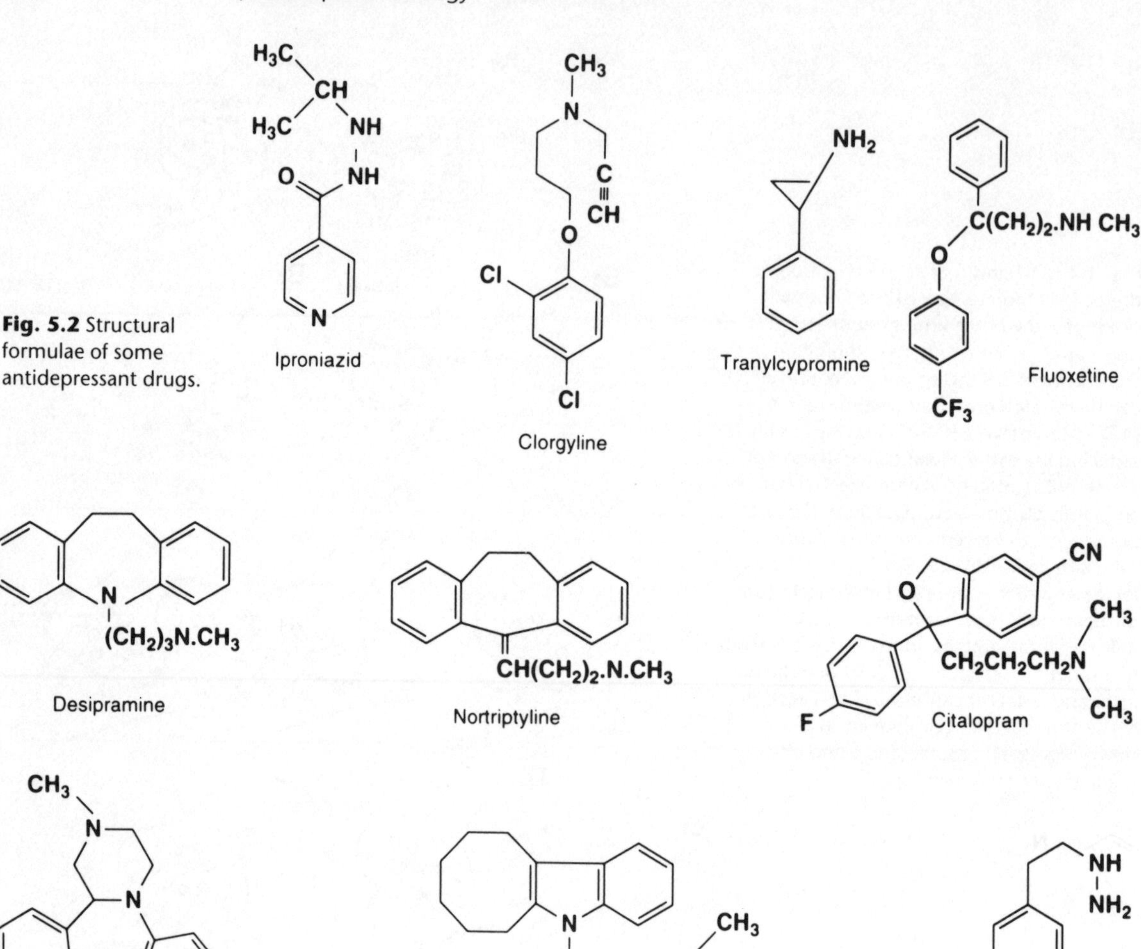


**Fig. 5.2** Structural formulae of some antidepressant drugs.

such 'suicide inhibitors' will take several days, until new MAO enzyme is synthesized by the cells.

## Problems associated with MAO inhibitors

The problems associated with the use of MAO inhibitors are many. Firstly, it may take 2 to 3 weeks before any sign of improvement in the psychological depression is seen, despite the relatively rapid inhibition of MAO activity and early increase of motor activity.

Secondly, many of the MAO inhibitors produce blockade of parasympathetic muscarinic receptors in the periphery leading to suppression of salivation, cycloplegia (loss of accommodation in the eye) and faecal/urinary retention. They can also produce chronic hypotension (due to the accumulation of 'false transmitter' amines which are less active than NA/NE in sympathetic nerve terminals) and an increase of food intake. They also have a net stimulant action

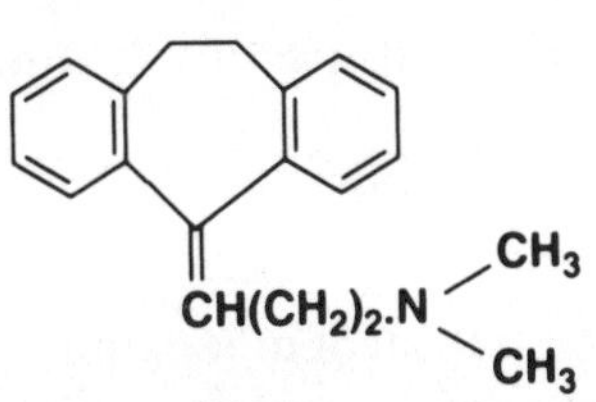

Amitriptyline

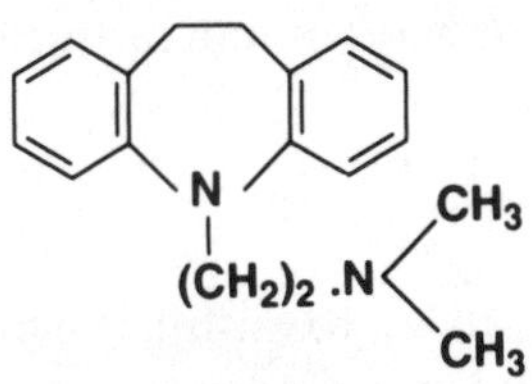

Imipramine

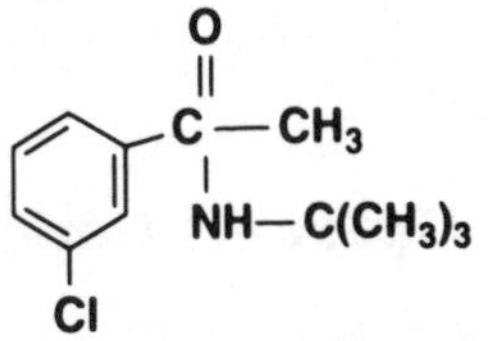

Bupropion

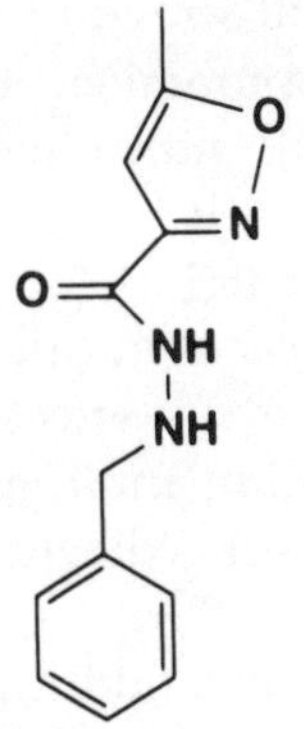

Isocarboxazid

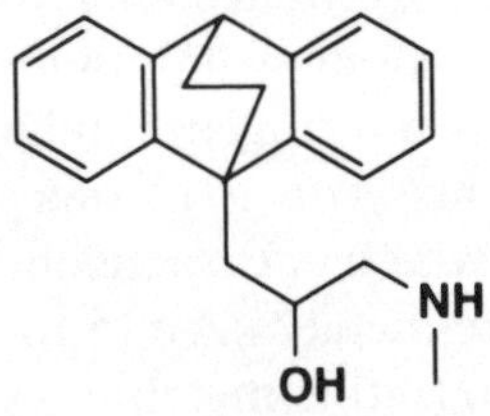

Oxaprotiline

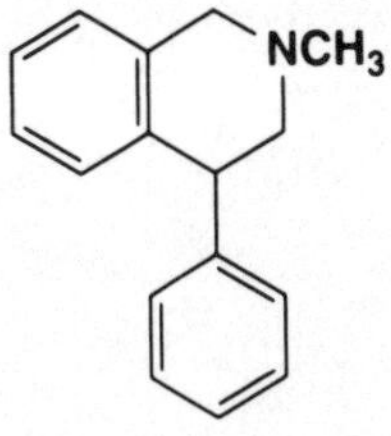

Nomifensine

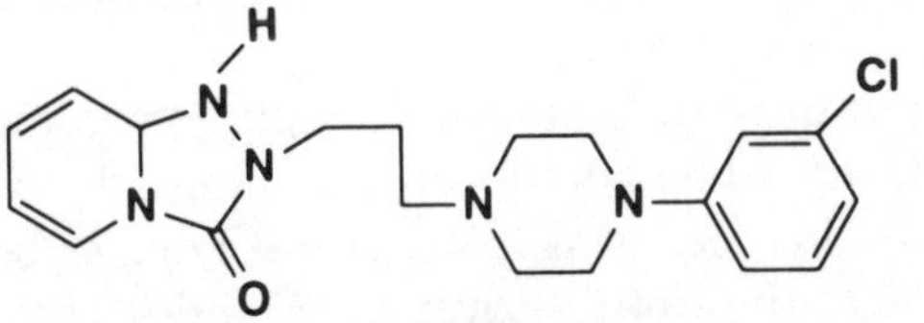

Trazodone

on the CNS which can result in restlessness, insomnia with a deficiency of REM sleep, delirium and tremors.

Thirdly, and perhaps most seriously, MAO inhibition can provoke the 'cheese reaction'. Some foodstuffs, including some cheeses, red wines, beans, beers, liver, bananas and fish contain tyramine and other phenylethylamine-derived, indirectly acting sympathomimetics (Chapter 3). These are normally destroyed by MAO in the intestinal wall, but following MAO inhibition their concentrations in the body can rapidly reach levels at which a massive displacement of NA/NE can take place from sympathetic nerve terminals, leading to a hypertensive crisis which can prove fatal. A similar potentiation will occur of indirectly acting amines such as ephedrine used in proprietary nasal decongestants. The half-life of other drugs metabolized by MAO will also be increased.

As noted above the non-specific MAO inhibitors are, because of these dangers, now less popular in clinical practice than 20 years ago. $MAO_A$ selective agents such as clorgyline are still useful since $MAO_B$ activity is sufficient to metabolize amines in the peripheral nervous system thus avoiding the cheese reaction. The persistence of muscarinic blockade and increased appetite remain, however.

## Uptake-1 inhibitors

An alternative approach to raising the functional concentration of monoamines in the extracellular space is to prevent the removal of released amines, which occurs by reuptake into the nerve terminals and varicosities (Uptake-1) (Figure 5.1B). The major drugs available with this property are the **tricyclic antidepressants** (TADs), so-called because their basic chemical structure consists of three adjacent rings (Figure 5.2). Secondary amines such as **desipramine** and **nortriptyline** show a preferential ability to inhibit the uptake of catecholamines, while their tertiary analogues **imipramine** and **amitriptyline** (with an extra methyl on the side chain nitrogen) inhibit mainly the removal of 5HT.

The tricyclics bind markedly to plasma proteins and can be displaced by other drugs such as aspirin which may therefore increase the incidence of side effects. The tricyclic drugs are metabolized in the liver by *N*-demethylation and ring-hydroxylation, though the metabolites produced retain pharmacological activity until they are eventually glucuronidated.

These compounds are very effective antidepressants and do not exhibit the cheese reaction. (Indeed they will prevent the action of indirectly acting sympathomimetic drugs such as amphetamine and ephedrine, and adrenergic neuron blocking drugs such as guanethidine because they will prevent the necessary uptake of these drugs into nerve terminals.)

The tricyclics do induce a number of unwanted effects, including postural hypotension due to some blockade of alpha-adrenoceptors, blockade of muscarinic receptors (dry mouth, blurred vision, constipation) and a degree of sedation. Some tolerance does develop to these effects over a few weeks. They also potentiate the depressant effect of ethanol on the CNS. This can be very marked and lead to death from respiratory depression. Probably the greatest danger with TADs is their ability to increase cardiac excitability, leading to dysrhythmias and potential heart failure.

As with MAO inhibitors there is also an uncomfortable latency of several weeks from starting drug treatment to the relief of depression, raising some doubts as to the relationship between MAO inhibition or Uptake-1 inhibition, and clinical improvement. These doubts are enhanced when it is realized that drugs such as amphetamine, which releases monoamines and inhibits uptake, or cocaine which inhibits uptake, have marked stimulant and euphoric effects on the CNS but do not relieve depression. (Chronic use of amphetamine leads to catecholamine depletion and induces depression!) As a result there is a continuing search for other neurochemical changes in depression, and for better, faster-acting drugs with fewer side effects.

### 5-Hydroxytryptamine

One result of research has been to shift the monoamine emphasis away from catecholamines and towards 5HT. There is a better correlation between the antidepressant activity of some drugs and their activity on 5HT containing neurons, than with their activity on catecholamine neurons. Inhibition of 5HT synthesis (using *p*-chlorophenylalanine, Chapter 4) can prevent the antidepressant activity of tricyclic antidepressants and MAO inhibitors. Furthermore, studies of the brains of depressed patients who have committed suicide reveal a decrease in the content of 5HT in several brain areas. There is also a loss of some 5HT receptors especially in the frontal cerebral cortex, but an increase in the number of $5HT_2$ receptors in some areas. This and related information had led to the introduction of compounds with a high selectivity for inhibiting the uptake of 5HT—drugs such as fluvoxamine, fluoxetine and citalopram (Table 5.1; Figure 5.2). Certainly a variety of antidepressant drugs as well as electroshock treatment for depression can enhance neuronal sensitivity to 5HT by increasing the number of $5HT_1$ and, particularly $5HT_2$ receptors. There is evidence that different drug classes affect these receptors at different sites, with MAO inhibitors reducing the number of presynaptic inhibitory receptors and TADs increasing receptor density postsynaptically. The net effect in both cases would be to facilitate 5HT-mediated neurotransmission.

The antidepressant drugs acting on amine uptake span a range for **citalopram** (Figure 5.2) with a greater than 5,000-fold selectivity for inhibiting 5HT uptake, through to **oxaprotiline** with a similar selectivity for NA/NE uptake—a range of 25 million. This emphasizes the difficulty in attributing antidepressant activity to interference with a single neuronal system.

## Atypical drugs

There are also a number of drugs which show very clear antidepressant activity, but their mechanism of action is uncertain; they do not seem to have particularly marked effects on the uptake or metabolism of catecholamines or 5HT, and are thus often referred to as atypical. They include **mianserin**, **iprindole**, **bupropion** and **nomifensine**.

Mianserin, iprindole and bupropion seem to have relatively little effect on catecholamine or 5HT uptake or metabolism and no effect on acetylcholine or histamine receptors. Mianserin does, however, block presynaptic $\alpha 2$-adrenoceptors (Figure 5.1c), preventing their normal inhibitory effect and leading to an increase of amine release. Nomifensine is rather unusual in that it very effectively inhibits the uptake of dopamine as well as NA/NE but has virtually no effect itself on 5HT. Its major metabolite, 4-hydroxynomifensine does, however, depress 5HT uptake. Both these compounds persist for a long time in the body, nomifensine having a half-life of around 24 hours, and its hydroxy derivative around 5 days. Nomifensine and bupropion have occasional serious side effects (hypersensitivity and convulsions, respectively) which have led to their withdrawal in some countries.

**Trazodone** has no effect on catecholamine systems but has activity, surprisingly, as a 5HT partial agonist, while at least one popular benzodiazepine, **alprazolam**, has antidepressant properties.

## A common mechanism?

In an attempt to find a mechanism of action which would be common to all antidepressant drugs, much recent research has been concentrated on the role of amine receptors. When a change occurs in the amount of transmitter available to act on its receptors, there is usually a compensatory adjustment by the cell in the number of receptors. An agent blocking receptors, for example, would lead to an increase in the number of receptors, an up-regulation, whereas some drugs, by increasing transmitter levels, might be expected to produce a decrease of receptor density—down-regulation. Since changes in receptor number imply changes at the level of gene regulation, it is expected that they might require several days to occur. In the case of antidepressants such a delay might help explain the long latency to the relief of depression.

### $\alpha$-Receptors

Several antidepressants, including particularly some of the atypical ones can rapidly block presynaptic $\alpha$2-adrenoceptors, thus removing their inhibitory effect on transmitter release (Figure 5.1C). The increased transmitter release in turn causes a long-term down-regulation in the number of $\alpha$2-receptors (Figure 5.1.C), and studies of amine effects on neuronal firing rates support this, with results showing a reduced sensitivity to NA/NE at $\alpha$2-receptors in the brain.

### $\beta$-Receptors

Most of the antidepressants can reduce the amount of cyclic AMP generated by stimulation of $\beta$-adrenoceptors. This is often, but not always, accompanied by a down-regulation in the number of $\beta$-adrenoceptors in the brain (Figure 5.1D) suggesting that in some cases $\beta$-receptors may be uncoupled from the adenylate cyclase system. These effects are seen with all classes of antidepressant, including some of those with selective effects on 5HT uptake (but not fluoxetine). It has also been shown that the use of $\beta$-receptor stimulant drugs, such as salbutamol and clenbuterol can have an antidepressant effect after only a few days. Some relationship may exist between $\alpha$- and $\beta$-adrenoceptor regulation since $\alpha$2-blockade can increase the down-regulation of $\beta$-receptors by antidepressant drugs. As noted earlier several typical and atypical antidepressants are able to increase the number of 5HT2 receptors (Figure 5.1D).

It is interesting that electroshock therapy, which is able to relieve depression even in patients showing little or no response to drugs, also results in a down-regulation of $\beta$-receptors. This change seems to occur in parallel with the antidepressant activity over about 2 weeks both in animal models and humans. There are also reports of an inherited overexpression of $\beta$-adrenoceptors in neurons and lymphocyctes of patients experiencing endogenous depression. The modulation of $\beta$-adrenoceptor number may, therefore, be a critical factor in the aetiology and treatment of depression.

Overall, the original simplistic Monoamine Hypothesis is being replaced by the 'dysregulation' hypothesis, which emphasizes the importance of a correct balance between all aspects of monoamine functions in the CNS and postulates that a disturbance at one of several points may lead to depression. Accordingly, pharmacological treatments may potentially involve interference at one of several sites.

# Mania

So far we have been concerned with patients suffering from depression only, so-called unipolar depression, but a small percentage of subjects experience bipolar depression or manic-depressive psychosis, in which the patient cycles between periods of profound depression and periods of hyperactivity and hyper-excitability with irritability, insomnia and impaired judgement. The patient now shows an inability to be still or quiet and may remain in this manic phase for hours or days before succumbing to another period of depression.

The most effective treatment for mania is the monovalent cation **lithium**, usually administered orally as lithium carbonate. Lithium has no effect in unipolar depression, but in manic-depressives it is able to suppress the mania ***and*** prevent the switch into the depressed phase. No-one really understands how lithium works. One hypothesis is that by replacing sodium to some extent it reduces neuronal excitability, neurotransmitter binding, and transmitter uptake which are often dependent on sodium concentration. The concentration of lithium achieved in the body, though, is only around 1 mmol/l and its effects may be more important in replacing sodium inside cells rather than outside where sodium concentration is around 120 mmol/l. Certainly lithium tends to accumulate inside cells and disturb membrane transport systems including the ATPase 'sodium pump'.

Lithium facilitates the uptake of NA/NE and 5HT and enhances the release of these and of acetylcholine. (The latter is particularly interesting since other cholinomimetics can also prevent mania.) Chronic treatment with lithium induces other changes of transmitter function, in common with other antidepressants, including a down-regulation of $\beta$-adrenoceptors. Lithium also enhances the release of 5HT from neurons and depresses the number of $5HT_2$ receptors. Interestingly, it also prevents the up-regulation of $D_2$ receptors seen following chronic neuroleptic therapy (Chapter 6).

Another possibility is based on the finding that lithium disrupts the cycle of phosphoinositide metabolism in cells. In particular, lithium blocks the resynthesis of PIP2 after its hydrolysis to IP3. Since the stimulation of this hydrolysis occurs in response to the activation of several types of receptor, this site of action would interfere with the effects of activating transmitter receptors, including muscarinic receptors for acetylcholine. Unfortunately lithium is quite toxic: its therapeutic concentration is around 1 mmol/l but above 2 mmol/l it can cause renal damage, mental confusion, seizures and coma.

Although not as effective as lithium, some neuroleptic drugs such as haloperidol (Chapter 6) are also able to control manic episodes, and they are far safer, and less toxic, than lithium. The anticonvulsant drug **carbamazepine** is also used as an antimanic agent and current research suggests that some benzodiazepines and calcium channel blockers may also be effective.

# 6 Psychotic disorders: neuroleptic drugs

## Introduction

The psychoses are those severe forms of psychiatric disorder in which the patient is usually unaware that s/he is ill. Patients lose contact with reality and exist in their individual and unique psychological world. (The distinction is often made from **neuroses** in which the patient is essentially normal except for relatively minor or specific personality or mental disturbances such as anxieties, obsessions or phobias).

The most common and best understood psychotic disorder is schizophrenia which affects about 1% of the population over the age of 20 years. In its early stages schizophrenia is characterized by a series of so-called Type I, positive or active symptoms, including (a) hallucinations; these are usually auditory and may involve voices of historical or religious characters, or may take the form of an independent voice commenting adversely on the patient's every action; (b) thought disorders; the patient is unable to think clearly and logically or to make simple deductions from a statement; s/he may instead make dangerously erroneous conclusions based on distorted logic; and (c) delusions; the patient's behaviour may be determined by a belief that they are a major political or religious figure, that they are being pursued or persecuted (paranoia) or even that people are intending to assassinate them. The patient may become a threat to other individuals as a result.

To some extent these early symptoms can be treated with the **antipsychotic** or **neuroleptic** drugs (formerly called major tranquillizers).

Unfortunately schizophrenia sometimes progresses to a stage in which behaviour is characterized by Type 2, or negative symptoms. The patient may withdraw totally from any contact or communication with other humans. In one extreme form patients may become catatonic; they will sit, stand, or crouch in one position, without moving, for hours on end. Some of these Type 2 patients show a flattening of affect; they may show no emotional response to major life events such as the death of a family member. Indeed, some patients exhibit inappropriate affective responses; they may laugh when told of a death or serious accident, and may show great distress when told of something amusing. These negative symptoms seem to correlate with a degeneration and shrinkage of the brain and enlargement of the cerebral ventricles. They are in general almost impossible to treat.

# Aetiology

One of the first clues to the mechanism of schizophrenia came from the realization that patients consuming amphetamines for several weeks or months, either as stimulants or appetite suppressants, could develop a disorder almost indistinguishable from schizophrenia—the amphetamine psychosis. Amphetamines produce a release of monoamines in the central as well as the peripheral nervous system. Conversely, if schizophrenic patients were given reserpine, which depletes monoamines in neurons, Type 1 schizophrenic symptoms were reduced. It has since been found that the most consistent change in post-mortem schizophrenic brains is an increased concentration of dopamine in the temporal lobe, especially the amygdala, and an increased number of dopamine receptors, especially D2 and D4 receptors (Chapter 4). There is some evidence for changes in the locus coeruleus and noradrenergic neurons, for 5HT involvement and most recently for a link between glutamate mediated transmission and schizophrenia. As yet there are no relevant antipsychotic drugs which affect selectively any of these transmitter systems, although compounds with quite selective properties as 5HT3 receptor antagonists are currently showing great promise in experimental test systems.

# Mechanism of action

Almost all the neuroleptic drugs now available are, in fact, dopamine antagonists. Figure 6.1 shows the remarkable correlation between the ability of drugs to displace radioactive ligands from dopamine receptors and the doses used clinically to suppress Type 1 schizophrenic symptoms.

Neuroleptics are thought to work at two sites on dopamine neurons. Firstly, they block postsynaptic D2 receptors on neurons of the mesolimbic pathway (Figures 4.4 and 6.2B). This is a very direct way of counteracting the presence of an increased number of receptors and a possibly increased release of dopamine.

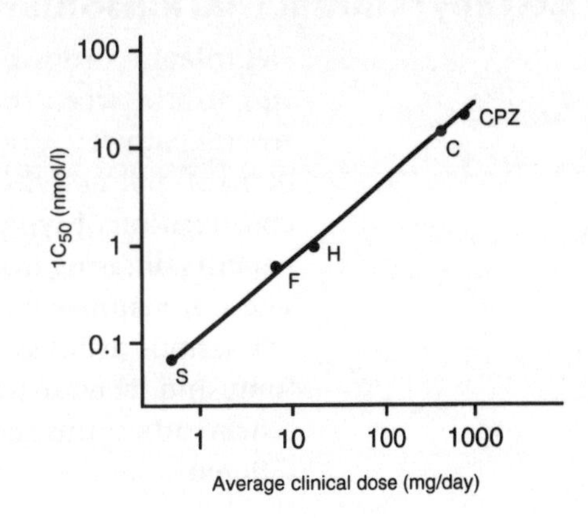


**Fig. 6.1** A graph illustrating the correlation between the clinical doses of neuroleptic (antipsychotic drugs) and their displacement of ligands from dopamine receptors. S, spiroperidol; F, fluphenazine; H, haloperidol; C, clozapine; CPZ, chlorpromazine.

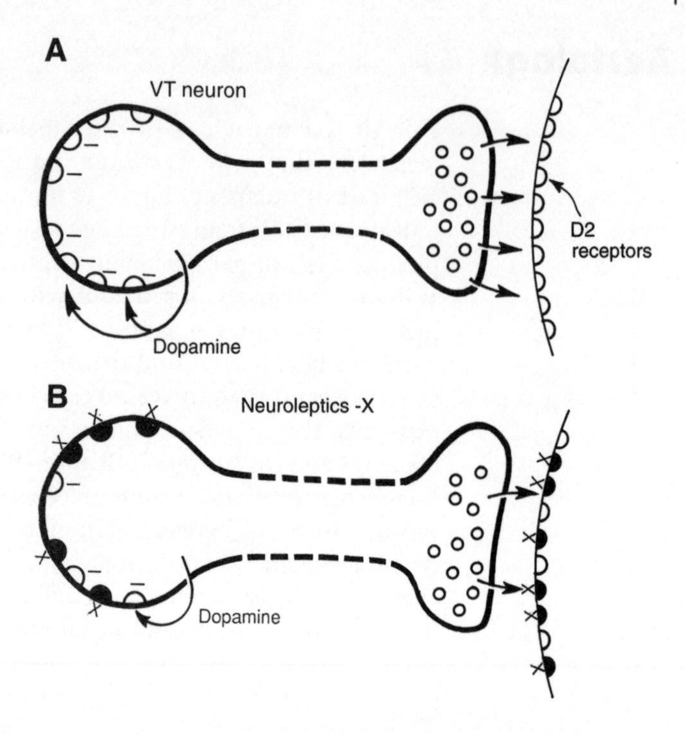


**Fig. 6.2** A neuron in the ventral tegmentum (VT) normally releases dopamine to act on postsynaptic D2 receptors in the limbic system and inhibitory autoreceptors on the cell bodies. (B) Neuroleptic drugs can block both types of receptor, preventing activation of target cells and causing over depolarization and inactivation of the dopaminergic neurons.

Secondly, the neuroleptics are able to block dopamine inhibitory autoreceptors located on the cell bodies of the mesolimbic neurons, in the ventral tegmentum (Figure 6.2B and Chapter 4). These are normally activated by dopamine released from the soma and dendrites or from recurrent branches of the ascending axons. By blocking these sites neuroleptics cause an initial increase of firing rate which leads to overdepolarization and thus inactivation after a couple of weeks. At this time the dopaminergic neurons, therefore, cease to fire and to release dopamine.

## Extrapyramidal (Parkinsonian) symptoms

Neuroleptic drugs possess one major disadvantage—most are unable to distinguish between the mesolimbic dopamine neurons and those in the nigrostriatal pathway. Consequently blockade of dopamine receptors and inhibition of neuronal activity will also occur in this pathway, leading to the same constellation of symptoms (tremor, rigidity, bradykinesia) seen in Parkinsonian patients suffering from a pathological degeneration of the pathway (Chapter 8). These are known as extrapyramidal symptoms (EPS) and are often reversible if neuroleptic drugs are withdrawn sufficiently quickly after their appearance. It is to try and increase the selectivity of drugs for mesolimbic neurons, as well as to reduce other unwanted effects such as sedation and hypotension that several different classes of neuroleptic drugs have been developed.

# Classes of drug available

## Phenothiazines

The phenothiazines were the first compounds used to treat schizophrenia and were developed after **chlorpromazine** (Figure 6.3) was introduced as an antihistamine and antiemetic, but was found to improve schizophrenic symptoms. It was later found to block dopamine receptors.

Phenothiazines

Phenothiazine nucleus

Aliphatic side chain:
Chlorpromazine:
$R_1$: $-(CH_2)_3.N(CH_3)_2$ $R_2$ : Cl

Piperazine side chain:
Fluphenazine:
$R_1$: $-(CH_2)_3.N$ [piperazine] $N(CH_2)_2.OH$ $R_2$ : $CF_3$

Piperidine side chain:
Thioridazine:
$R_1$: $-(CH_2)_2$ [N-methylpiperidinyl] $R_2$ : $SCH_3$

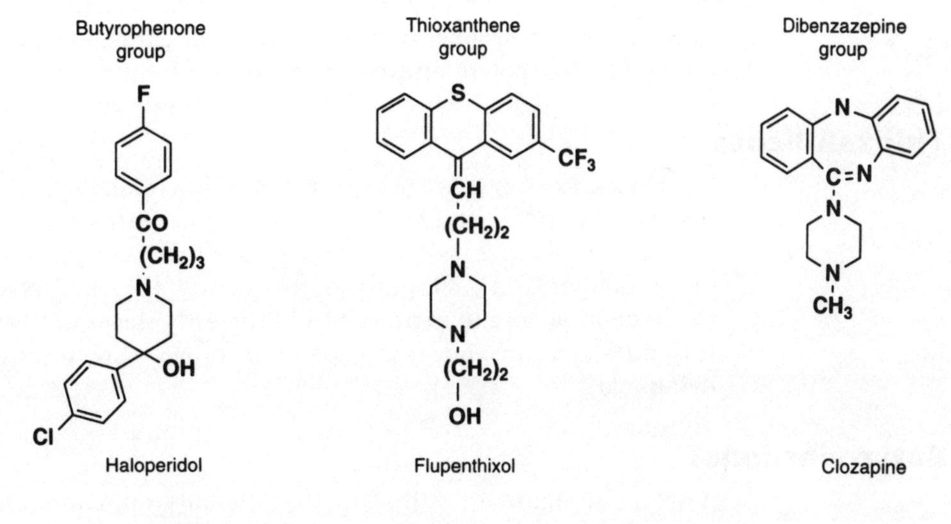


**Fig. 6.3** Structural formulae of some neuroleptic drugs.

Pimozide

Sulpiride

There are several subtypes of phenothiazines depending on whether the side-chain (R1 in Figure 6.3) carries an aliphatic (straight-chain) grouping (chlorpromazine), a piperazine grouping (fluphenazine) or a piperidine group (thioridazine).

The aliphatic group of drugs tend to be rather non-selective, blocking peripheral receptors for acetylcholine (muscarinic), NA/NE (alpha), 5HT and histamine (H1) as well as dopamine. This results in a plethora of side effects, including postural hypotension, dry mouth, blurred vision and constipation.

One of the most marked CNS side effects is sedation, probably due to the block of muscarinic and histamine receptors. This may, of course, be advantageous in hyperactive or aggressive patients. The antiemetic effect of these drugs may also be useful and is due to the blockade of dopamine D2 receptors in the chemoreceptor trigger zone in the hindbrain.

The piperazine phenothiazines are generally more potent than the above and show much less block of non-dopamine receptors. They are consequently much less sedative. Both aliphatic and piperazine derivatives can induce marked Parkinsonian (extrapyramidal) symptoms.

The piperidine derivatives have sedative properties intermediate between the other phenothiazines. They are also less likely to block $\alpha$-adrenoceptors, 5HT or histamine but they retain appreciable potency as central muscarinic antagonists. Since Parkinsonism can be treated with muscarinic antagonists (Chapter 8) the piperidine phenothiazines carry an in-built anti-Parkinsonian defence which means fewer patients develop Parkinsonian symptoms on these drugs. All phenothiazines are able to potentiate the depressant effects of ethanol on the CNS to a potentially dangerous degree.

## Thioxanthenes

The thioxanthenes (e.g. flupenthixol) are structurally very similar to the phenothiazines and resemble the piperazine phenothiazines in pharmacology. They are less sedative than any of the phenothiazines but show greater blockade of central muscarinic receptors. Consequently, they are less likely than any of the phenothiazines to produce EPS in the early stages of treatment. However, this does not preclude some patients progressing to irreversible tardive dyskinesia.

## Butyrophenones

A glance at Figure 6.1 will show that the butyrophenones (e.g. haloperidol) resulted from a search for dopamine antagonists with high potency and selectivity. While this certainly eliminates most of the interference with peripheral autonomic function and most of the sedation, it also removes the safety feature of central muscarinic blockade (Chapter 8). Some patients are, therefore, more likely to develop Parkinsonian symptoms than on previous drugs. In practice schizophrenic patients are often started on butyrophenones because of their selectivity and later switched to other drugs if they begin to develop Parkinsonism.

## Atypical neuroleptics

In addition to the drugs discussed above there are several groups of compounds which are far less likely to produce EPS and are, therefore, known as 'atypical' antipsychotics. They include diphenylbutylpiperidines (pimozide), benzamides (such as sulpiride) and dibenzodiazepines (clozapine) (Figure 6.3). This last drug is worth discussing in more detail.

### Clozapine and D4 receptors

Clozapine (Figure 6.3) has been regarded as the most effective drug treatment for schizophrenia. The reason for its efficacy is not certain because it has relatively poor affinity for D2 receptors (Figure 6.1) and also blocks D1 receptors. There is some evidence though, that 5HT pathways may be involved in schizophrenia and clozapine is able to block $5HT_2$ and $5HT_3$ receptors as well as dopamine receptors.

There has been much excitement recently with the discovery that additional types of dopamine receptor exist in the CNS, notably a D3 and a D4 subtype and that, in human brain tissue, clozapine shows a 10-fold higher affinity for these sites than for other dopamine receptors. This raises the possibility that schizophrenia may involve an over-expression of D4 receptors and that clozapine's effectiveness results from its selectivity for this site. The localization of D4 sites to the mesolimbic system also helps explain the relative absence of EPS with clozapine. In addition, clozapine has marked central antimuscarinic properties which help preclude EPS and it is also very unlikely to produce tardive dyskinesia (see later).

So why is clozapine not our major antipsychotic drug? Unfortunately it had to be withdrawn in 1984 because a few patients developed fatal blood disorders such as agranulocytosis. It has only recently been reintroduced for patients refractory to other drugs; blood from these patients is screened every two weeks and treatment is stopped if any signs of leucocyte depletion are detected.

## Side effects of antipsychotic drugs

The tendency of some drugs to induce autonomic dysfunction by blocking muscarinic receptors (reduced salivation, cycloplegia, faecal and urinary retention, increased intraocular pressure) or alpha-adrenoceptors (postural hypotension) has been mentioned previously. Sedation due to block of central muscarinic and histamine receptors is also common and EPS have been mentioned as a major problem.

Another consequence of blocking dopamine receptors is the emergence of hyperprolactinaemia with breast development in both sexes. This results from blockade of receptors normally responsible for inhibiting the release of prolactin from the anterior pituitary.

### Tardive dyskinesia

A further problem is that when some patients have been treated with neuroleptic drugs for several years, they may develop tardive (slowly developing) dyskinesias (motor abnormalities). These usually involve the face and mouth and are seen mainly as continuous movements of the lips, mouth and tongue. It is generally believed that they result from an up-regulation of dopamine receptors as a compensation for the blockade of receptors by the neuroleptic drugs. However, withdrawal of the drugs does not stop the dyskinesias, i.e. they are usually irreversible, and a recent alternative theory is based on an apparent degeneration of strionigral and other striatal output neurons containing GABA. This would remove inhibitory control of pallidal and thalamic neurons involved in movements and lead to the release of involuntary movements.

## Sigma receptors

Another recent development has been that some potent antipsychotic agents such as haloperidol can bind with high affinity to a non-dopamine receptor referred to as the sigma site (because it also binds some opiate-like compounds such as pentazocine which were once considered to act on a sigma-opiate receptor; there is in fact no functional relationship between sigma sites and opiates or analgesia). The role of these haloperidol-sensitive sigma receptors is a mystery, and it is not known whether there is a natural, endogenous ligand for them. Nevertheless, haloperidol derivatives with selective effects at sigma sites are being developed as possible future neuroleptic drugs.

# 7 Sedatives and anxiolytics

## Introduction

In general, drug treatments for sleep and anxiety disorders are similar. Some authorities indeed define sedative drugs as those which reduce anxiety, and hypnotics as those which promote sleep, but the terms anxiolytics and sedative/hypnotic drugs, respectively, are to be preferred since they make the rationale for their use clearer, and some drugs are able to reduce anxiety without producing significant sedation.

## Sleep

Most people sleep for about 8 hours each day, with a sleep phase which consists of alternating periods of rapid eye movement (REM) and non-REM sleep. Non-REM sleep itself consists of four stages (I–IV) characterized by an EEG of progressively lower frequency and high amplitude (delta waves). Stage IV sleep represents a deep sleep which the brain attempts to recoup first after a period of sleep deprivation. Periods of REM sleep, which last for about 10–30 minutes at a time, recur every 90 minutes or so, and represent the periods during which dreaming is thought to occur. The brain tries to recover REM sleep also with a high priority after deprivation.

It has been estimated that one third of adults seek help for some form of sleep disturbance at some time. Sedative drugs (hypnotics if they induce sleep at high doses) are used to reduce the latency to the onset of sleep and to prolong the period of continuous sleep, thus assisting the brain to achieve adequate Stage IV and REM sleep.

## Anxiety

Everyone is anxious, worried, about something at some time. For reasons which are not clear, some people experience much more profound and prolonged anxiety, often out of all proportion to what they may claim as the precipitating factor(s). This can lead to severe headaches, profuse sweating, aggression, depression, and an inability to concentrate on work. In some patients these symptoms may occur without any obvious physical cause and without any evident triggering factors.

Some extreme forms of anxiety are very specific, and take the form of phobias such a as agoraphobia (fear of open spaces) and its opposite claustrophobia (fear of enclosed spaces). Acute reactions to these situations are often referred to as panic attacks, but they appear to respond better to antidepressant drugs (Chapter 5) than to anxiolytics.

# Drugs used as sedatives or anxiolytics

## Barbiturates

Barbiturates are now largely of historical importance, some having been formerly used as long-acting sleep-promoters and anxiolytics. They do, however, cause an initial reduction of REM sleep and, if administration is stopped suddenly, a large rebound increased of REM sleep. This can be associated with especially vivid, nightmarish dreams which can cause further insomnia or anxiety, as a result of which the patient seeks to return to the drug. In addition, physical dependence can develop, so that abrupt withdrawal from barbiturates results in nausea and vomiting, anxiety, hallucinations and convulsions. Barbiturates are thus considered addictive and, given that they also cause marked respiratory depression, daytime 'hangover' sedation, induction of liver enzymes etc. (see Chapter 8) they have largely been superseded by benzodiazepines. Indeed the only barbiturate still prescribed (rarely) for sedation is **pentobarbitone** (**pentobarbital**) (Figure 7.1). Tolerance occurs to the sedative activity relatively quickly, within 10–14 days. This is only partly due to the induction of liver microsomal enzymes (which are responsible for the metabolism of barbiturates and many other classes of drug), and is primarily a functional tolerance since tolerance to other effects such as respiratory depression appears more slowly. This presents the hazard, especially with the elderly, of patients increasing the dose of pentobarbitone, and/or repeating the dose on waking early, only to die from probable respiratory depression due to overdosing.

## Benzodiazepines

The benzodiazepines form a large class of compounds in which a variety of substitutions are present on a basic tricyclic structure (Figure 7.1). Among the most common ones in clinical use are **triazolam**, **lorazepam**, **chlordiazepoxide**, **nitrazepam**, **flurazepam** and **diazepam**. They differ widely in their duration of action, the examples just listed having plasma half-lives of around 4, 12, 15, 30, 40 and 50 hours, respectively. Oxazepam ($t_{1/2}$ around 10 hours) is an active metabolic product of several benzodiazepines.

Although different members of the benzodiazepine series find use as sedatives or anxiolytics, anticonvulsants or muscle relaxants, individual members of the group have some degree of selectivity. As sedatives, for example, nitrazepam, temazepam and flurazepam are preferred while diazepam, lorazepam and

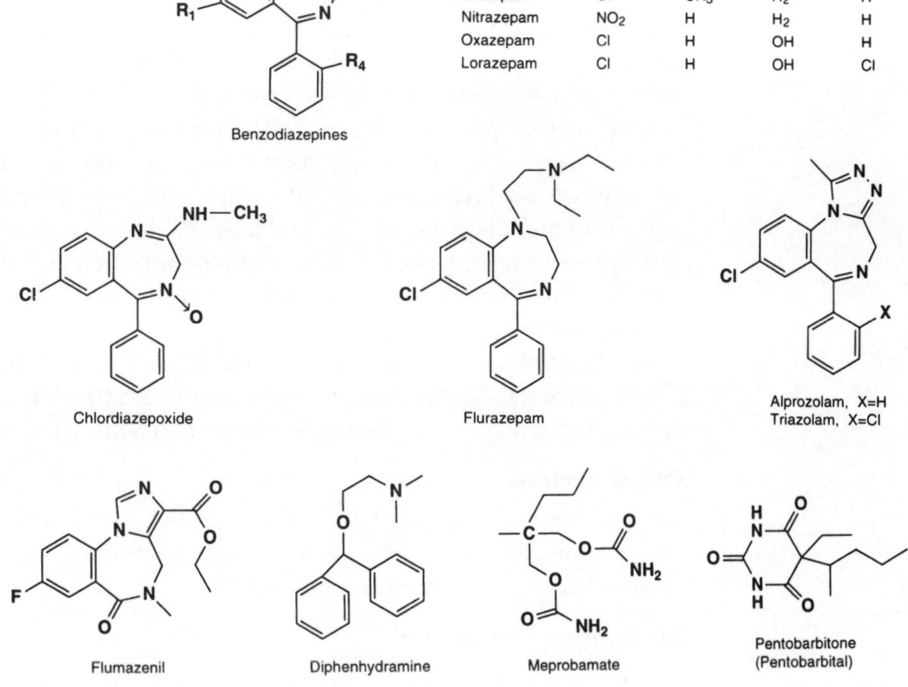


| | R1 | R2 | R3 | R4 |
|---|---|---|---|---|
| Diazepam | Cl | $CH_3$ | $H_2$ | H |
| Nitrazepam | $NO_2$ | H | $H_2$ | H |
| Oxazepam | Cl | H | OH | H |
| Lorazepam | Cl | H | OH | Cl |

**Fig. 7.1** Structural formulae of sedative drugs including a series of benzodiazepines.

chlordiazepoxide are more effective as anxiolytics. (Midazolam is used for anesthetic induction and clonazepam as an anticonvulsant.) In most patients tolerance develops to the sedative, muscle relaxant and anticonvulsant activities of benzodiazepines, but not to the anxiolytic effects.

Benzodiazepines cause few unwanted side effects when taken at correct dosage levels. There is also a benzodiazepine antagonist available, **flumazenil**, which can be injected to facilitate arousal of patients after overdosing and prevent excessive depression of the CNS. Occasionally patients may exhibit a paradoxical aggression on benzodiazepines. Mild confusion and drowsiness, with slight motor incoordination early in treatment may present problems if driving, or the operation of complicated machinery is important to the patient's work. In elderly subjects the mild confusion may exacerbate the declining mental alertness of age, and could be mistaken for dementia. All benzodiazepines potentiate the depressant activity of ethanol. Triazolam has received attention recently after reports that chronic administration was associated with violent psychotic episodes. However, it appears to be a useful short-acting drug ($t_{1/2}$ = 3 hours), and can rapidly induce both profound sedation and amnesia. It can produce marked rebound confusion.

For many years it was believed that cessation of benzodiazepine administration was not associated with any clear withdrawal symptoms. It is now recognized, however, that about 25% of patients treated with high doses of these drugs for long periods (3 months or longer) will experience headaches, insomnia, increased anxiety, dizziness and nausea on cessation of treatment especially if the drugs are withdrawn rapidly. These symptoms are generally not serious, and are easily mistaken for a mild bout of influenza, hence the delay in recognizing them as a drug withdrawal syndrome.

One of the greatest dangers with benzodiazepines is that patients may become psychologically dependent on them. The mild calming, anxiolytic activity is one which some patients, consciously or unconsciously, find advantageous in their daily hectic, stressed lives. While some people obtain relaxation through exercise or moderate intake of ethanol, there is a widespread tendency for some patients to achieve the same objective by continued administration of benzodiazepines.

All benzodiazepines are lipid soluble and cross the blood–brain and blood–placental barriers easily. They are metabolized by hepatic microsomal enzymes, but do not induce any increase of enzyme activity.

### Other actions

Because benzodiazepines have an overall inhibitory action on the CNS (see later), some members of this group are very useful as anticonvulsants (page 94) or as centrally acting muscle relaxants.

### Mechanisms of action

The main means by which benzodiazepines are believed to exert all their actions — anxiolytic, sedative, anticonvulsant, muscle relaxant — is by enhancing the inhibitory activity of GABA at $GABA_A$ inhibitory synapses. One possible explanation for this variety of effects is that there are at least three different benzodiazepine binding sites — BZ1, BZ2 and BZ3 (occasionally known as $\omega$ (omega)-1, $\omega$2, $\omega$3) distinguished on the basis of distribution and pharmacology. The last of these occurs mainly in peripheral tissues and in the mitochondria of glial cells in the CNS and its function is unknown. The BZ1 site occurs mainly in the hippocampus and BZ2 mainly in the cerebellum. Clinically used benzodiazepines may affect these various sites differently. There may also be a large variety of subtly different ways in which benzodiazepines could modify GABA (or $\beta$-carboline etc.) activity, depending on the precise subunit composition of the GABA receptor: the receptor consists of two to five subunits from a large selection. There appears to be a high affinity binding site for the benzodiazepines on the $\gamma$-subunits of the $GABA_A$ receptor, quite distinct from the GABA binding sites on the $\beta$-subunits (Figure 7.2). Receptors consisting of $\alpha 1 \beta 1 \gamma 2$ subunits exhibit BZ1 pharmacology, while receptors containing any of the $\alpha 2$ to $\alpha 6$ subunits show BZ2 pharmacology.

The attachment of a benzodiazepine to its binding site causes an allosteric change in the $GABA_A$ receptor such that GABA binding is enhanced (an **allosteric** change is one mediated by complex molecular interactions involving changes of receptor conformation, in this case between two different receptor subunits). The affinity ($K_d$) of GABA for its receptor is increased, but not the

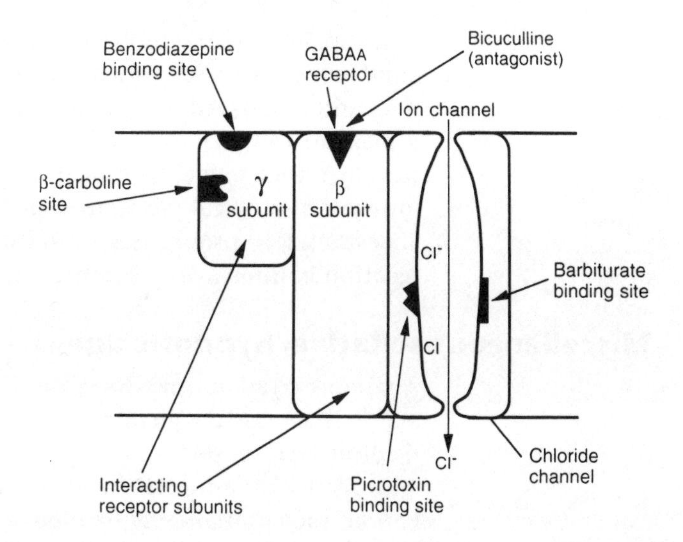


**Fig. 7.2** The GABA receptor/channel complex includes binding sites for GABA itself, on the $\beta$-subunit. These can be blocked competitively by bicuculline. The $\gamma$-subunit has binding sites for benzodiazepines and $\beta$-carbolines. The chloride channel which is opened by GABA receptor activation has binding sites for picrotoxin (a channel blocker) and barbiturates (increasing channel opening).

number of receptors ($B_{max}$). The net result is to increase the number of chloride channels opened by GABA at one time (sometimes stated as an increase in the frequency of opening) thus causing an increase of neuronal inhibition. (Note the distinction from barbiturates, Chapter 8, which prolong the duration of opening of individual channels.) The receptor interaction is a mutual one — GABA also increases the affinity of benzodiazepines for their binding sites.

### Endogenous ligands?

The benzodiazepine binding sites are something of a mystery. There have been suggestions that they may be receptors for endogenous GABA-modulating peptides (GABA-modulin and diazepam-binding inhibitor) and even that the brain produces its own benzodiazepines! Benzodiazepine-like molecules in the brain of drug-naive subjects, however, may originate in the diet or as a result of metabolizing dietary constituents.

One class of compounds which is known to exist in the brain and affect benzodiazepine sites are $\beta$-carbolines. These are products of 5HT condensation with alcohols or aldehydes. Some synthetic $\beta$-carbolines bind to benzodiazepine sites but have the opposite effect of decreasing GABA function. They are therefore known as inverse agonists. They produce, or increase, anxiety rather than reduce it, and lower the threshold for seizures rather than raise it. It is fascinating to speculate on whether anxiety is dependent on the presence of endogenous $\beta$-carbolines and that the anxiolysis by benzodiazepines results from their antagonism. Flumazenil blocks the effects of $\beta$-carbolines as well as of benzodiazepines.

Finally it should be remembered that some effects may be produced only indirectly. Suppose that anxiety, for example, involved a primary disturbance of 5HT neurons (see later); an increased GABA inhibition of those neurons might lead to a compensatory up-regulation of 5HT receptors, which relieves the problem.

It should again be emphasized that the benzodiazepines are in use not just as anxiolytics but also as anticonvulsants (Chapter 8), and muscle relaxants, sedatives and for anaesthetic induction. Their popular use as premedication before general anaesthesia results from their ability to reduce patient apprehension and to reduce skeletal muscle tone for surgery. They are used to provide sedation for unpleasant medical procedures such as endoscopy, or operations under local anaesthesia, to provide sedation during dental procedures and for prolonged sedation in intensive care units.

## Miscellaneous sedative/hypnotic agents

A number of additional drugs are available for use as sedatives, though in general they are not as well tolerated as benzodiazepines, and their use needs closer medical supervision.

Several histamine H1 receptor antagonists which cross the blood–brain barrier, such as **diphenhydramine**, will produce marked sedation. (This is often an unwanted side effect of the use of these drugs to suppress motion sickness, an action which is probably related more to the central muscarinic receptor blockade produced than to any effect on histamine receptors; the sedative effect may be partly due to histamine blockade.)

There is also a miscellaneous group of compounds including **meprobamate**, **methaqualone**, and **paraldehyde** which have sedative activity. Although still in use (paraldehyde or chloral hydrate can be given rectally in small children) they have been largely superseded for adults by benzodiazepines.

$\beta$-Adrenoceptor antagonists, or $\beta$-blockers such a propranolol (Figure 3.9) are said to penetrate into the brain and reduce anxiety. Most of their usefulness probably arises from their blockade of peripheral sympathetic activity which can cause laryngeal tenseness, increased cardiac activity (palpitations) and hand tremor. By preventing these obvious signs of nervousness, the $\beta$-blockers make the subject feel better subjectively and increase self-confidence. A true sedative/anxiolytic action of propranolol on the CNS may occur but has been attributed to the isomer which does not block $\beta$-adrenoceptors.

## Anxiety and 5HT related drugs

Agonists at $5HT_{-1A}$ receptors show anxiolytic activity in animal models. Several such compounds, such as **buspirone** are being introduced into clinical practice for the treatment of anxiety, since the anxiolytic action is not accompanied by sedation or motor problems. Anxiolysis is not seen for 1 or 2 weeks, however, raising the possibility, as with the antidepressants, that indirect effects may be responsible. These might include inhibition of 5HT neurons or neurons possessing $5HT_{1A}$ receptors, and a compensatory up- or down-regulation of non-5HT receptors.

# 8 Movement disorders

## Introduction

Humans are afflicted by a variety of serious motor disorders, some of which cannot currently be treated with drugs. Amyotrophic lateral sclerosis (ALS or motoneurone disease) involves a progressive loss of spinal and cortical motoneurons, resulting in initial clumsiness progressing to total paralysis in some patients. The cause of neuronal death is unknown, although recent evidence suggests that excessive activation of kainate receptors by glutamate (Chapter 4) or the presence of free radicals such as $OH^{\bullet}$ may be involved. Although there is research into the possible use of thyrotrophin analogues, kappa opiates, gangliosides, growth factors and lamotrigine as therapeutic agents, there is presently no effective drug treatment.

## Multiple sclerosis

Multiple sclerosis is an autoimmune disease in which the body produces antibodies that cause a patchy destruction of the myelin sheath surrounding large diameter axons. The result is slowed conduction causing a range of neurological symptoms including clumsiness which can develop into an incapacitating degree of spasticity. Research is primarily aimed at improving axonal conduction in the early phases of the disease. Compounds such as the aminopyridines block the outward potassium current which contributes to axonal repolarization. Consequently the action potential becomes broader (more prolonged), allowing spikes to 'jump' several segments of demyelinated axon and helping to maintain conduction velocity.

## Parkinson's disease

Parkinson's disease was first described by James Parkinson in London in 1817. It is characterized by three primary symptoms: (a) a coarse, slow tremor (3–5 Hertz), mainly visible in the hands; (b) muscular rigidity, which causes patients to adopt a flexed posture and to show little facial expression; and (c) bradykinesia (or hypokinesia). Partly because of (a) and (b) patients tend to make few movements and move very slowly. They have difficulty initiating movement and, later in the disease, may be forced to stand or sit immobile for long periods until able to move further. Once moving, patients have difficulty stopping.

The disease usually appears after about 60 years of age and appears to be due primarily to degeneration of dopaminergic neurons in the pars compacta of the substantia nigra which normally project to the neostriatum (the nigrostriatal tract, Chapter 4). There is also a marked loss of noradrenergic neurons in the locus coeruleus and 5HT releasing neurons in the raphe nuclei. The disease is usually idiopathic (i.e. of unknown causes). As first discovered by Hornykiewicz in 1960, there is a decrease of striatal dopamine content to 20% or less of control brains, with a corresponding decrease of the dopamine metabolite homovanillic acid (HVA) in the cerebrospinal fluid. The involvement of this particular pathway is supported by the fact that reserpine (which depletes neuronal catecholamines, Chapter 3) and neuroleptic drugs (which block dopamine receptors, Chapter 6) can induce Parkinsonian symptoms (often called extrapyramidal symptoms, EPS). Severe Parkinsonism has also been produced in drug addicts who inadvertently consumed the toxic compound 1-methyl-4-phenyl-1,2,3,6-tetrahydropyridine (MPTP). This agent is oxidized by monoamine oxidase-B to a metabolite which is taken up selectively by dopaminergic neurons and subsequently causes their death.

It is not surprising then that most drug treatments are designed to compensate specifically for the loss of dopaminergic neurons. Dopamine itself cannot be given because it does not cross the blood–brain barrier, but its synthetic precursor, Dopa, is an amino acid which is carried across the vascular endothelium by amino acid transporters (Figure 8.1).

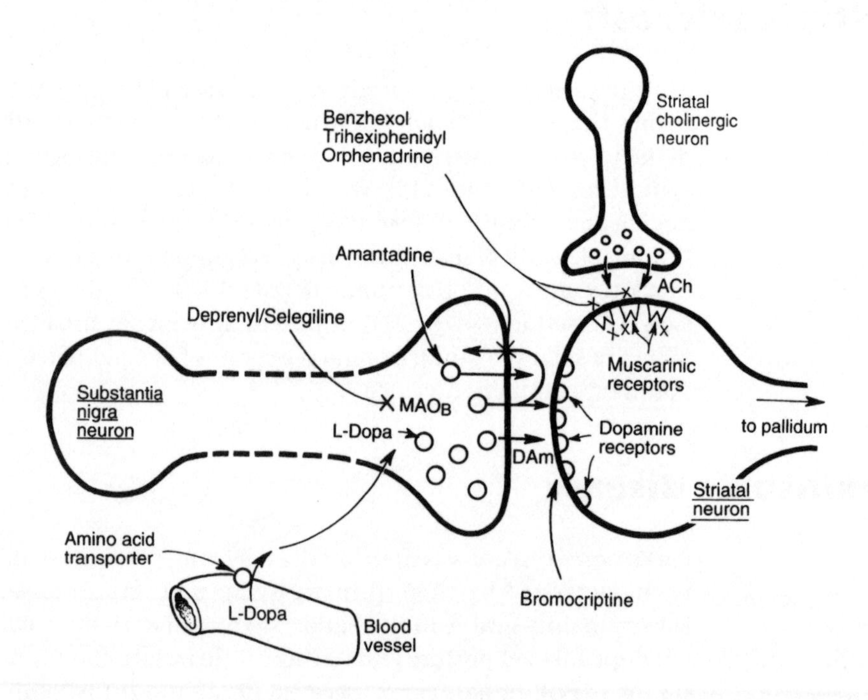


**Fig. 8.1** Sites of action of drugs affecting nigrostriatal dopaminergic neurons.

## L-Dopa (levodopa)

The most effective agent for Parkinson's disease is L-dopa (the L-isomer of 3,4-DihydroxyPhenylAlanine), usually known as **levodopa** (Figure 8.2). Dopa is a component of the normal biosynthetic pathway for dopamine (Chapter 4) and the administration of large doses of L-dopa alone (2–10 grams/day) seems to increase the amount of dopamine synthesized in the brain. The conversion may take place in some noradrenergic and 5HT-releasing neuron terminals as well as surviving dopaminergic ones.

One of the biggest problems with levodopa is that around 99% of an oral dose is metabolized by L-aromatic amino acid decarboxylase (dopa decarboxylase) in the intestinal walls, plasma and tissues. In practice therefore dopa is now administered together with compounds which inhibit this enzyme peripherally, but which cannot themselves penetrate into the brain. The two major inhibitors of peripheral dopa decarboxylase are **carbidopa** (Figure 8.2) and **benserazide**. The combination of levodopa with one of these raises the cerebral bioavailability of oral L-dopa from 1% to around 10% so that the dosage can be reduced by about 75%. Attempts are continuing to develop selective peripheral inhibitors of the other amine metabolizing enzyme, catechol-*O*-methyltransferase (COMT) which should raise bioavailability further to around 60%.

The administration of levodopa can produce a truly dramatic improvement in Parkinsonian patients. Patients who are seated or bed-ridden, virtually unable to move, dress or feed themselves are transformed after an hour or so into apparent normality, walking around and behaving as if normal. Unfortunately this apparently miracle treatment does not provide the full answer for Parkinsonian patients. As the degeneration of the nigrostriatal neurons progresses, with the loss of aromatic amino acid decarboxylase in the striatum, so levodopa becomes less and less effective. For many patients it is virtually ineffective after several years of the disease. In addition, many patients experience very disconcerting on–off, effects, in which the effectiveness of the drug seems to fluctuate rapidly. A patient may move around normally, then sit down and find 5 minutes later that s/he is unable to sit up. Yet another 20 minutes or an hour later s/he will carry on as normal. The cause of on–off effects is unknown but is probably related to the pharmacokinetics of L-dopa: on–off effects are much less evident if the drug is administered by intravenous infusion, and seem to be worse in the periods following meals, probably due to competition between dietary amino acids and L-dopa transport carriers into the brain. Another way of avoiding the phenomenon where it is a major problem is to use the dopamine agonist apomorphine, which can be administered by injection continuously, or as required by the patient.

Two other side effects of levodopa therapy are interesting in other contexts. Firstly, prolonged treatment can result in a schizophrenia-like syndrome in some patients. The development of these symptoms is interesting in view of the belief that true schizophrenia is itself caused by excess dopaminergic activity (Chapter 6).

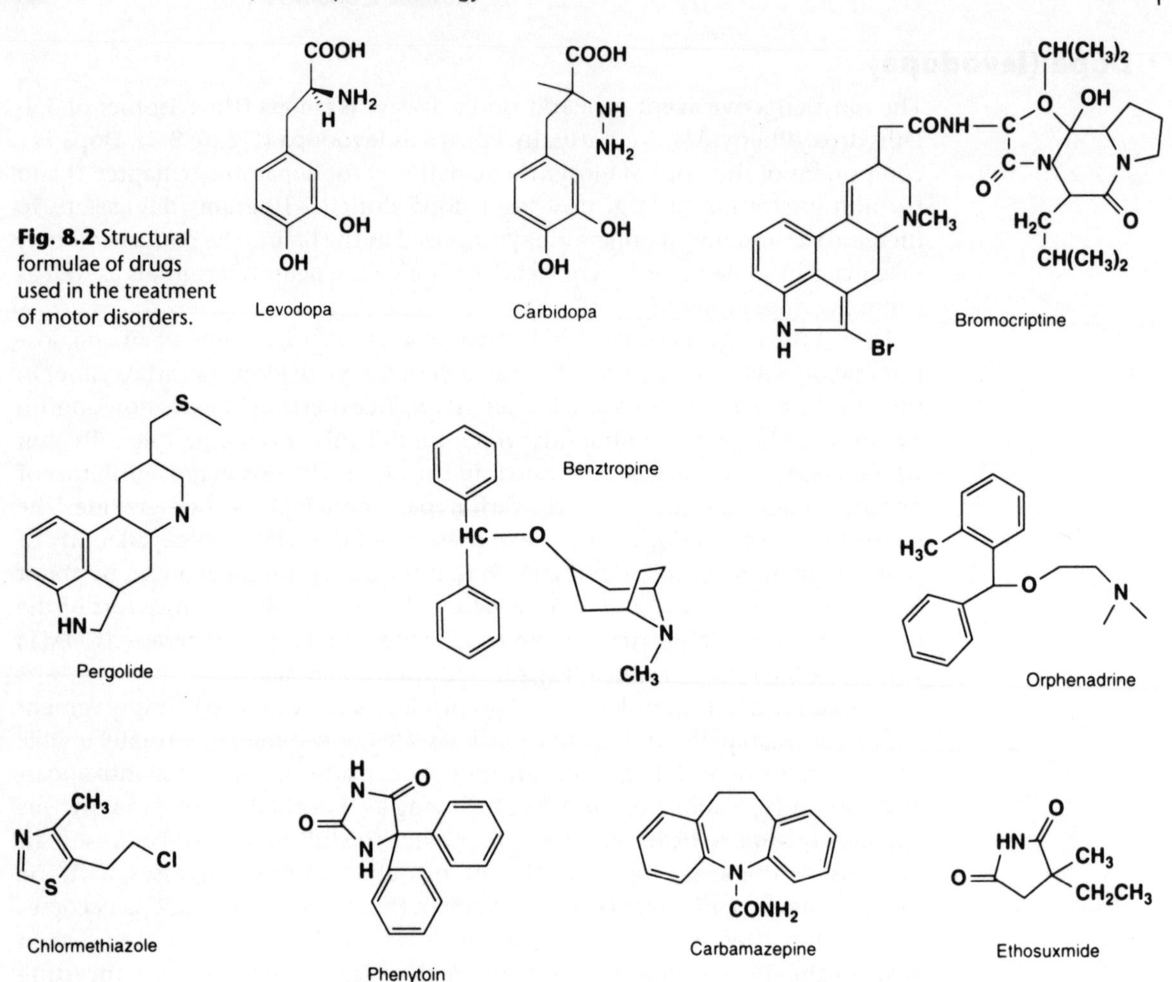


**Fig. 8.2** Structural formulae of drugs used in the treatment of motor disorders.

Secondly, prolonged treatment with levodopa can lead to the emergence of new involuntary movements such as athetosis (slow, writhing, snake-like movements) and choreiform movements (rapid, jerky, twitch-like). Some of these movements resemble those of Huntington's chorea, to be discussed later.

Both the psychiatric and movement difficulties can develop to the extent that they are severely incapacitating, and some patients may even prefer the difficulties associated with the Parkinsonian symptoms to the side effects of L-dopa.

In the early phase of treatment with levodopa many patients experience nausea (due to stimulation of dopamine receptors in the chemoreceptor trigger zone of the medulla oblongata), cardiac dysrhythmias (due to stimulation of $\beta$-adrenoceptors by dopamine) and hypotension (due to the dilution of transmitter NA/NE in sympathetic nerves by inactive 'false transmitter' metabolites of dopa and dopamine). The nausea tends to disappear after a few weeks and can also be prevented by the peripheral dopamine antagonist domperidone.

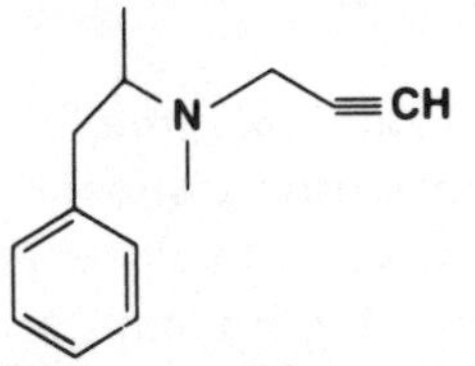

Deprenyl (Selegiline)

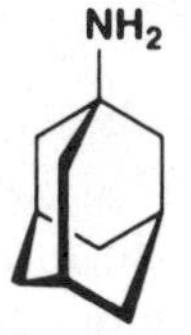

Amantadine

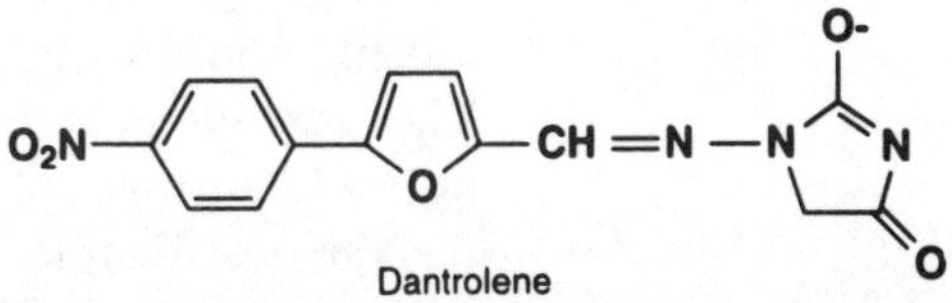

Dantrolene

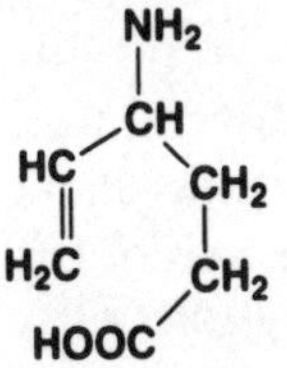

Vigabatrin

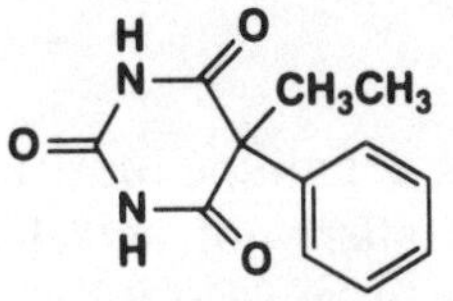

Phenobarbitone (phenobarbital)

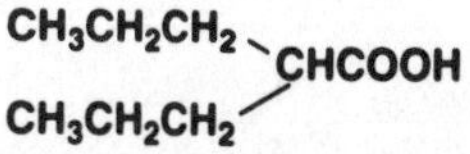

Valproic acid

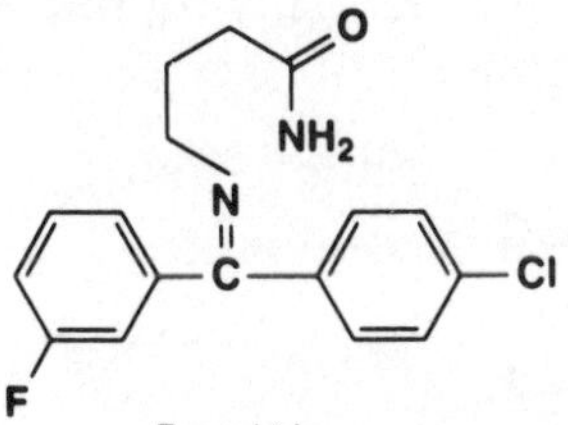

Progabide

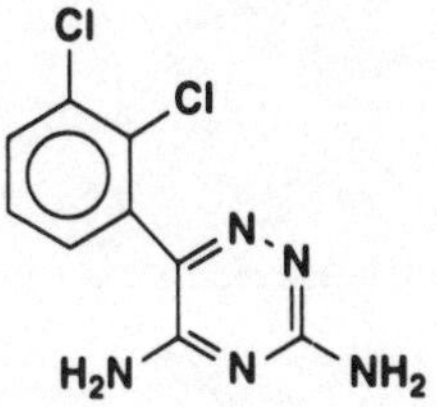

Lamotrigine

## Deprenyl (selegiline)

Deprenyl is a selective inhibitor of $MAO_B$, the predominant form of MAO in human brain, and the isozyme primarily responsible for the oxidation of dopamine. Deprenyl alone can increase dopamine levels in the brain sufficiently to treat early, mild cases of Parkinson's disease, and is often used with levodopa to enhance its efficiency. There is also recent evidence that deprenyl may even slow down the rate of nigrostriatal degeneration.

## Amantadine

Amantadine was first used as an antiviral drug and found accidentally to improve the mobility of Parkinsonian patients. It is now known to promote the release of dopamine from intact neurons and to inhibit the uptake of dopamine. Like levodopa therefore, it is only effective in the presence of some dopaminergic terminals, and is now little used. Its use in early Parkinsonism, however, can delay the need for levodopa and, in turn, delay the possible onset of psychiatric (schizoid) side effects.

## Bromocriptine

There are several drugs which act as directly acting agonists at dopamine D2 receptors and which have been shown to be effective in Parkinson's disease. They include **bromocriptine, pergolide** and **lisuride**. They are of particular use in the later stages of the disease when dopaminergic degeneration is complete but the postsynaptic receptors remain. One side effect of these ergot alkaloids is their suppression of pituitary prolactin release due to the activation of hypothalamic receptors for dopamine (that is, prolactin release inhibitory factor). However, this is not a major clinical problem.

## Anticholinergic drugs

The inhibitory effects of dopamine on striatal neurons are normally counterbalanced by excitatory effects of acetylcholine released from intrastriatal interneurons and acting on muscarinic receptors (Figure 8.3). The loss of the nigrostriatal pathway thus leaves an excessive unbalanced cholinergic activity. By suppressing this with muscarinic antagonists, the symptoms of Parkinsonism can be controlled and many clinicians begin therapy of mildly affected patients with amantadine or anticholinergic drugs in order to delay the need for L-dopa. Several anticholinergic drugs are available which act preferentially on mus-

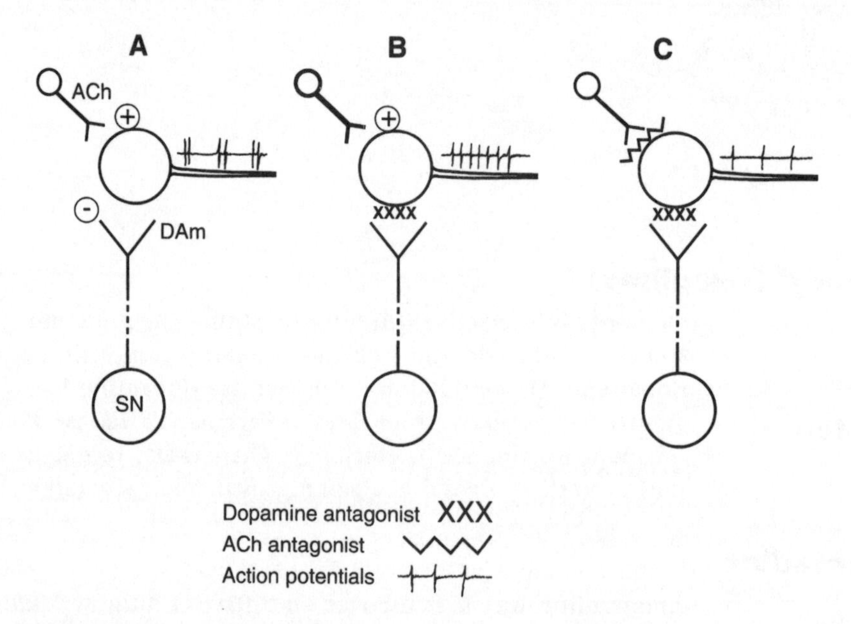


**Fig. 8.3** Properties of neuroleptic drugs. (A) In the normal brain, the effects of the inhibitory (-) dopaminergic nigrostriatal pathway are balanced by excitatory (+) cholinergic neurons within the striatum. Blockade of dopamine receptors by neuroleptic drugs (X) can result in the relative overactivity of the cholineric input, causing Parkinsonian symptoms (B). If a neuroleptic drug has some ability to block muscarinic receptors, it will reduce the cholinergic stimulation and prevent the extrapyramidal disorders, (C).

carinic receptors in the CNS, and thus do not produce excessive problems with peripheral parasympathetic blockade. These drugs include **benztropine**, **trihexiphenidyl**, **procyclidine** and **orphenadrine**. They may cause some drowsiness and may enhance confusion in the elderly, in whom they are now rarely used.

## Huntington's disease (chorea)

The jerky, choreiform (dance-like) movements of the hereditary disorder Huntington's disease are similar to those produced in some Parkinsonian patients by levodopa therapy. Indeed the problem seems to lie in an uncontrolled dopaminergic tone in the basal ganglia, probably due to the loss of GABA releasing inhibitory interneurons. Levels of dopamine in Huntingtonian striata are normal, but there is a profound loss of GABA and its synthetic enzyme GAD (Chapter 4). Drugs which activate dopaminergic neurons or receptors therefore make Huntington's patients worse, and the best treatments are dopamine antagonists (Chapter 6) or anticonvulsant benzodiazepines. Some features of the disease can be reproduced in animals with toxins such as quinolinic acid which destroys GABA-containing neurons. Since quinolinic acid is normally present in the brain it, or a related compound, may be involved in the aetiology of this disease. In most patients the striatal neurodegeneration is followed by cortical degeneration leading to dementia.

## Spasticity

Following damage to the motor areas and pathways of the brain there is often an increased tone of skeletal muscle, and this rigidity results in severe deficits of motor movement and coordination. This state is known as spasticity. The most effective treatment is with drugs which act on the CNS to produce a decreased tone of skeletal muscle by suppressing activity in polysynaptic excitatory pathways.

### Baclofen

**Baclofen** (Figure 4.7) is an agonist at the $GABA_B$ population of receptors and causes both direct inhibition of interneurons and a diminution in the release of excitatory transmitters such as glutamate. The GABA transaminase inhibitor **vigabatrin** (Figure 8.2) raises the CNS level of GABA and is effective in controlling spasticity. **Benzodiazepines** are also useful, probably because they also enhance inhibitory tone in the CNS (Chapter 7) and cause muscle relaxation.

Another drug which can be used in spasticity is **dantrolene**, although this acts not on the nervous system but directly on muscle to reduce the release of calcium for contraction from the sarcoplasmic reticulum.

# Epilepsy

The major disorders involving seizures or convulsions are the epilepsies. They affect 0.5–1% of the population and may be idiopathic (cause unknown) or a result of cerebral disorders such as tumours, CNS infections or stroke. Epileptic attacks seem to begin as an abnormal, excessive firing of a group of neurons referred to as the trigger or focus. The disease may take various forms including:

(a) simple partial, or Jacksonian, in which motor movements originate in a restricted part of the body and gradually spread to other parts of the body;

(b) complex partial, or psychomotor in which there may be sudden affective (mood) changes accompanied by complex rhythmic stereotyped movements which appear to be purposeful (e.g. repeatedly stroking a hand or combing the hair),

(c) generalized tonic–clonic, in which movements may originate locally but soon the entire body is involved in a tonic–clonic convulsion—the tonic phase implies rigidity in the muscles, giving way to the clonic phase involving violent spasmodic contractions of the limb and facial musculature; patients lose consciousness during these episodes. If prolonged, as status epilepticus, there is the danger of suffocation, respiratory failure, serious brain damage, or even death in 10% of cases.
EEG records (high voltage, high frequency, often with a spike and wave format) can often be used to support the diagnosis of these epilepsies and to localize the trigger focus. (Correct diagnosis is essential since many disorders such as panic, sleep difficulties, abnormal respiration or some forms of poisoning can result in seizures which may be made worse by drugs used in epilepsy!)

(d) absence seizures, sometimes known as petit mal episodes do not involve convulsions, but are transient lapses of consciousness. The patients, usually children, are often unaware that they have been effectively unconscious for several seconds and carry on as if nothing had happened. The episodes may be detected clinically by monitoring the associated EEG changes (high voltage, low frequency). These episodes, if frequent, can be very disruptive of a child's education: the experience must be like listening to a lecture where the microphone repeatedly goes dead for 10 or 15 seconds at a time.

## Drugs used in epilepsy

Drugs used in epilepsy are given in Figure 8.2 and Table 8.1.

### Benzodiazepines

The benzodiazepines have been discussed earlier in relation to their sedative and anxiolytic properties (Chapter 7), but several of these compounds are useful in the treatment of some epileptic disorders. Among the most commonly used are clonazepam, lorazepam and diazepam, the latter often being the drug of choice, administered by injection for the rapid termination of status epilepticus.

**Table 8.1** Drug therapy of motor disorders

| Disorder | Drugs | Mechanism |
|---|---|---|
| Multiple sclerosis | Aminopyridines | Block $K^+$ channels and speed axonal conduction |
| Parkinson's disease | L-dopa (+ carbidopa or benserazide) | Precursor of dopamine (inhibitors of peripheral dopa decarboxylase) |
| | Amantadine | Release dopamine Inhibits dopamine uptake |
| | Deprenyl (selegiline) | MAO-B inhibition |
| | Bromocriptine | D2 receptor agonist |
| | Trihexiphenidyl Benztropine Orphenadrine Procyclidine | Muscarinic receptor blockers |
| Huntington's disease | Benzodiazepines (diazepam) | Potentiate $GABA_A$ inhibition |
| | Neuroleptics | Block dopamine receptors |
| Spasticity | Benzodiazepines | Potentiate $GABA_A$ inhibition |
| | Baclofen | $GABA_B$ agonist |
| | Mephenesin | Blocks postsynaptic reflexes |
| Epilepsy | | |
| Partial–simple or complex (psychomotor); Generalised tonic–clonic | Carbamazepine | Use-dependent block of $gNa^+$ |
| | Phenytoin | Use-dependent block of $gNa^+$ |
| | Phenobarbitone (phenobarbital) | Potentiation of $GABA_A$ |
| | Primidone | Potentiation of $GABA_A$ |
| | Valproate | Potentiation of $GABA_A$ and increase of GABA levels. |
| | Vigabatrin | Inhibits GABA transaminase |
| Absence seizures | Valproate | Potentiation of $GABA_A$ and increase of GABA levels |
| | Ethosuximide | Unknown |
| | Clonazepam | Potentiation of $GABA_A$ |
| Status epilepticus | Diazepam | Potentiation of $GABA_A$ |
| | Chlormethiazole | Possible potentiation of $GABA_A$ |

## Hydantoins

Hydantoins such as **phenytoin** (5,5-diphenylhydantoin) are frequently used as antiepileptic drugs for simple partial seizures. Phenytoin has a relatively low therapeutic index and can cause a variety of side effects including vertigo, confusion, insomnia, ataxia and megaloblastic anemia. Most troublesome is the fact that its metabolizing enzymes are saturated at therapeutic plasma levels. Elimination thus follows zero order kinetics and small changes in dosage can produce wide fluctuations in plasma concentrations with the possibility of accumulation to toxic levels. It is thus important to consider the ability of many drugs such as cimetidine and valproate to inhibit hepatic metabolizing enzymes, potentially causing dramatic increases in the plasma concentration of phenytoin, and leading to signs of toxicity. Phenytoin, like the barbiturates to which it is chemically related, is an inducer of hepatic microsomal enzymes.

### Mechanism of action

Phenytoin has many properties in common with the local anaesthetics, and can block sodium channels in a use-dependent fashion. It is thus able to stabilize the neuronal firing, producing a disruption of activity in those neurons firing rapidly in the epileptic focus, while having little effect on neurons firing at more normal frequencies. In addition, phenytoin is able to enhance activity of the sodium/potassium (ATPase) pump, thus reducing further the excitability of neurons experiencing a large influx of sodium due to excessive firing. The drug has also been found to inhibit calcium-dependent calmodulin protein kinases, which are thought to be involved in neurotransmitter release.

## Carbamazepine

Carbamazepine is becoming increasingly popular as an anticonvulsant as it is relatively non-toxic. Its main metabolite, carbamazepine-10,11-epoxide also possesses anticonvulsant activity. The 10-keto analogue of carbamazepine, **oxcarbazepine**, is being developed as an alternative to the parent drug, with reportedly fewer side effects.

### Mechanism of action

Carbamazepine resembles phenytoin in blocking sodium channels and thus producing a local anaesthetic-like stabilization of neurons trying to fire rapidly during epileptic activity.

## Valproate

The sodium salt of valproic acid is one of the most effective agents for the long-term control of tonic–clonic and other seizures. Because it causes little sedation and is relatively non-toxic, it is especially useful in the treatment of children.

### Mechanism of action

Valproate is believed to act partly like phenobarbitone, increasing the duration of chloride channel opening in response to GABA activation, and partly by increasing the synaptic concentrations of GABA in the CNS. This in turn may be the result of inhibiting GABA-transaminase and succinic semialdehyde dehydrogenase, the two enzymes, mainly responsible for the metabolism of GABA.

## Vigabatrin

Vigabatrin is a simple derivative of GABA, gama-vinylGABA. It is a potent suicide inhibitor of GABA transaminase (i.e. it forms a covalent bond with the enzyme, from which neither the drug nor the enzyme recover).

## Ethosuximide

Ethosuximide is one of the few drugs which is selectively useful against absence seizures; it can even precipitate, tonic–clonic convulsions in susceptible individuals. Although related structurally to barbiturates its mechanism of action is unknown.

### Chlormethiazole

Chlormethiazole is one of the few drugs which, like diazepam, can be given intravenously to interrupt status epilepticus. It stops the seizures very rapidly, probably by enhancing GABA-mediated inhibition, though the detailed mechanism is not known.

### Barbiturates

Barbiturates are substituted derivatives of barbituric acid, with a wide range of properties depending on the nature of the substituents. **Phenobarbitone** (phenobarbital) (Figure 8.2) has a relatively useful ratio of anticonvulsant activity to sedative activity and is the only barbiturate routinely used in epilepsy, although pentobarbitone is of use in refractory status epilepticus. Like all barbiturates, phenobarbitone produces marked respiratory depression and is an inducer of hepatic microsomal metabolizing enzymes. The metabolism of the barbiturate itself is thus increased, as well as of many other drugs such as oral contraceptives, dexamethasone, vitamin D, $\beta$-blockers, tricyclic antidepressants, anticoagulants etc., and dosage of these needs to be increased accordingly. Conversely, dosage needs to be corrected downwards following barbiturate withdrawal. Withdrawal can also lead to insomnia, anxiety, hypotension, delirium and seizures. Patients will naturally try to avoid these withdrawal symptoms by continuing to take barbiturates when no longer necessary—they are seriously addictive. As CNS depressants, barbiturates will potentiate ethanol, leading to coma and possible respiratory arrest.

The enzyme $\delta$-aminolaevulinic acid synthase is one of the enzymes induced by barbiturates and in susceptible patients the increased formation of porphyrin precursors can exacerbate acute porphyria, causing abdominal pain, photosensitivity, vomiting, confusion and paralysis, which can be life-threatening.

#### Mechanism of action

The barbiturates enhance the ability of the inhibitory neurotransmitter GABA to open chloride channels in the neuronal membrane. The drugs bind to a site associated with the channel itself rather than to the GABA receptor, with the result that the channel, once activated by the $GABA_A$ receptor complex remains open longer, i.e. the duration entry and neuronal hyperpolarization. The barbiturate binding site is related to the site at which the GABA antagonist picrotoxin acts to block chloride movement through the channel (see Figure 7.2). In addition barbiturates are also able to block receptors for the excitatory transmitter glutamate, especially the population site sensitive to AMPA (Chapter 4).

### Primidone

If the oxygen atom on the 3-carbon of phenobarbitone (phenobarbital) is removed, there results a deoxybarbiturate—primidone. Primidone is metabolized partly to phenobarbitone in the body and its pharmacology is therefore very similar, though it is overall less potent and induces fewer serious side effects.

Table 8.1 summarizes the categories of epilepsy and the drugs usually considered the most appropriate treatments.

## Drugs of the future

Since none of the drugs presently available is ideal there is still a great deal of effort expended trying to develop improved compounds. These include: (a) GABA prodrugs such as **progabide** which penetrates into the CNS where it is hydrolysed to yield GABA and thus cause inhibition of neuronal firing; (b) inhibitors of GABA uptake such as **tiagabine**; (c) GABA analogues such as **gabapentin**; (d) calcium channel blockers such as **flunarizine**, which reduces neuronal excitability and transmitter release; (e) glutamate antagonists—experimental compounds that block NMDA receptors and show promise as anticonvulsant drugs; and (f) inhibitors of glutamate release from neurons, such as **lamotrigine**.

# 9 Analgesics

## Introduction

Pain is often a warning that tissue damage is being produced and that the causative agent or action should be removed or stopped. Pain often continues after the removal of the stimulus, possibly as a reminder that the injury needs attention; it also accompanies chronic inflammatory conditions such as arthritis, it is triggered by some tumours (mechanism unknown) and it may appear to arise in an amputated limb (phantom pain). In all these cases it may be difficult for patients to carry on normal lives without the use of drugs to suppress or at least control the pain.

## Drugs affecting sensory receptors

Following acute tissue damage, as with a cut or knock to the skin, a variety of cellular components gain access to the extracellular fluid. These include adenosine, adenosine triphosphate (ATP), 5HT, histamine and bradykinin. Soon after injury macrophages and cells of the immune system invade the damaged area in an attempt to remove cell debris and to prevent or combat any infection by microorganisms. Activation of the immune cells leads to the activation of phospholipase A2 and the formation of eicosanoids (20-carbon metabolites of arachidonic acid, such as prostaglandins). These in turn are released into the extracellular space and, among other things, sensitize nociceptive nerve endings in the tissue to compounds such as histamine and bradykinin. The resulting stimulation of these afferents gives rise to the perception of pain.

One means of suppressing the pain is to suppress the immune system and the production of prostaglandins with, for example, glucocorticoids. In order to distinguish them from glucocorticoids, another group of compounds which affect nociceptive afferent stimulation are known as the non-steroidal anti-inflammatory drugs (NSAIDs).

### NSAIDs

#### Mechanism of action

Basically, NSAIDs suppress the formation of prostaglandins from arachidonic acid, and thus remove the sensitizing action which these lipids have on noci-

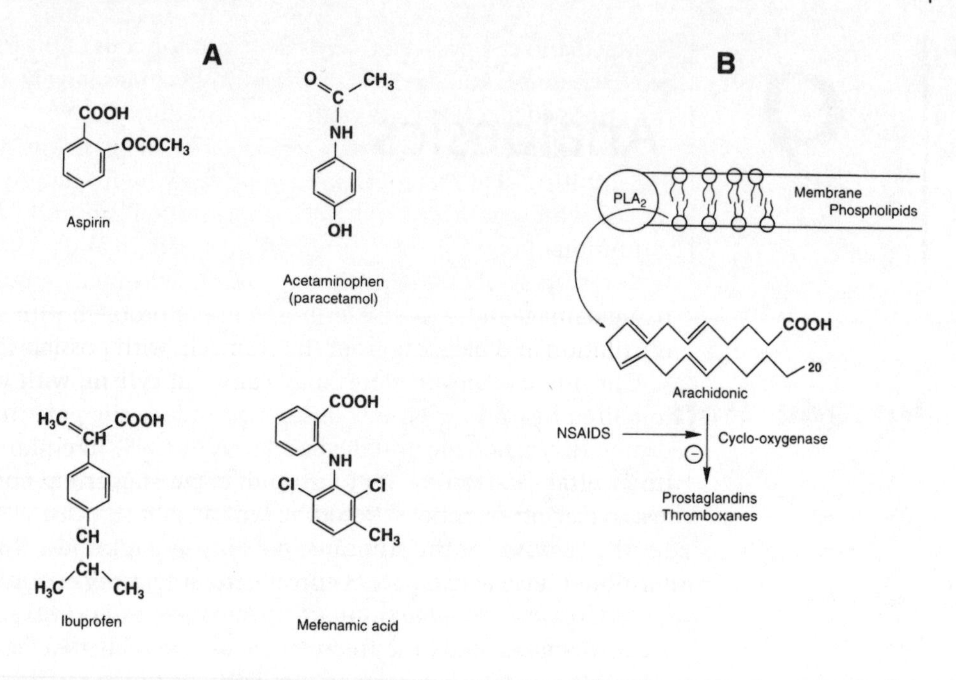


**Fig. 9.1** (A) Structural formulae of some non-steroidal anti-inflammatory drugs (NSAIDs). (B) NSAIDs act by preventing the conversion of arachidonic acid into prostaglandins and thromboxanes. Arachidonic acid is split off from membrane lipids by phospholipase A2 (PLA2).

ceptors. Of the various NSAIDs available, **aspirin** (acetylsalicylic acid) (Figure 9.1) is the best known.

## Aspirin

Aspirin inhibits cyclo-oxygenase, the enzyme responsible for the synthesis of prostaglandins and thromboxanes from arachidonic acid (Figure 9.1B). Aspirin produces an irreversible acetylation of the enzyme so that recovery requires synthesis of new enzyme which takes several days. Other NSAIDs have a less permanent action. The inhibition of cyclo-oxygenase produced by **indomethacin** is reversible when the drug is removed, and a similar, competitive inhibition is produced by **piroxicam** and phenylpropionic acids (**ibuprofen** etc.) which compete with the normal substrate arachidonic acid.

The mechanism of action of **acetaminophen** (paracetamol) is not entirely understood. Although it does inhibit cyclo-oxygenase, it is much weaker than aspirin. This may explain the lack of anti-inflammatory activity and the absence of aspirin-like side effects such as gastric bleeding and impaired coagulation, but how then does it produce analgesia? It has been suggested that acetaminophen may have more activity in the CNS and that the weak inhibition of eicosanoid metabolism in the CNS has a disproportionate effect on pain perception. It is also possible that the drug interferes with other aspects of nociceptive afferent stimulation at the site of tissue damage. Recent evidence indicates that acetaminophen may act to reduce the levels of endogenous lipid peroxides which normally promote activity of the cyclo-oxygenase enzyme.

## Unwanted effects of salicylates

Aspirin binds to plasma proteins and can displace other drugs. As it is an acid a significant proportion (about 99%) is un-ionized in the acid medium of the stomach and can pass relatively easily into the cells of the gastric wall. Inside the cells, where pH is nearer 7.4, the aspirin becomes largely ionized (99.99%) and thus trapped at a relatively high concentration.

Prostaglandins are normally produced by the gastric wall and have the effect of inhibiting acid secretion and promoting the formation of the thick layer of mucus which helps protect the gastric epithelium from the high acidity. The inhibition of prostaglandin production by aspirin and other salicylates (see later) thus results in increased acid and decreased mucus production—a recipe for tissue damage in the gastric lining. A major problem with salicylates, therefore, is irritation and bleeding from the stomach, with possible formation of ulcers.

Chronic use of salicylates may cause salicylism, with vertigo, tinnitus and impaired hearing. Even low doses may induce the potentially fatal Reye's syndrome (liver damage and degeneration of CNS) in children with influenza or other viral infections. The inhibition of prostaglandin and thromboxane synthesis (see later) will also affect blood coagulation since thromboxane release from platelets is an important factor in aggregation; bleeding time may be increased several-fold for around 10 days after a singe dose of aspirin.

Whereas the salicylates, including aspirin, reduce inflammation as well as the pain associated with it, it may often be appropriate to diminish the pain but not the inflammation. In those cases phenacetin or its active metabolite acetaminophen (paracetamol) may be used. In fact phenacetin has no advantages over acetaminophen but is considerably more toxic; it is no longer used clinically.

### Acetaminophen

Acetaminophen (paracetamol), on the other hand, is remarkably safe and induces few unwanted effects at normal doses. Its main danger is in overdosage, when a toxic, highly reactive metabolite (*N*-acetyl-*p*-benzoquinone) can accumulate in the liver and kidney and cause serious irreversible and occasionally fatal tissue damage.

### Other NSAIDs

A group of phenylpropionic acids includes **ibuprofen**, **ketoprofen** and **naproxen**. Their adverse effects are generally similar to aspirin, with gastric bleeding and increase bleeding time. The related group of phenylacetic acids such as **diclofenac** have similar unwanted effects. The fenamates include **mefenamic acid** and **meclofenamate**. These can still cause serious gastrointestinal distress, as can the chemically unrelated drug piroxicam.

A number of compounds with structures based on the indole nucleus are also available including **indomethacin** and **sulindac**. They are used more for their anti-inflammatory activity than for analgesia, as are some pyrazolone compounds such as **phenylbutazone**.

## Centrally acting analgesics

Centrally acting analgesics are listed in Table 9.1. These are drugs often related to **morphine**, the major active constituent of the poppy secretion known as opium. They are therefore known generically as **opiates** or opioids, the former

**Table 9.1** Analgesic drugs

| Peripherally acting (NSAIDs) | Centrally acting (opioids) |
|---|---|
| Aspirin (a salicylate) | Morphine ($\mu$ agonist) |
| Acetaminophen (paracetamol) | Meperidine (pethidine) ($\mu$ agonist) |
| | Methadone ($\mu$ agonist) |
| Ibuprofen (a phenylpropionic acid) | Fentanyl ($\mu$ agonist) |
| Mefenamic acid (a fenamate) | Buprenorphine ($\mu$ partial agonist) |
| Phenylbutazone (a pyrazolone) | Pentazocine ($\mu$ partial agonist, $\kappa$ agonist) |
| Diclofenac (a phenylacetic acid) | Butorphanol ($\mu$ antagonist, $\kappa$ agonist) |
| | Nalorphine ($\kappa$ agonist) |
| | Naloxone ($\mu > \kappa$ antagonist) |

term being preferred for compounds showing clear structural similarities with morphine, while the term opioids may include a variety of dissimilar chemicals, including endogenous neuropeptides, with actions that resemble those of morphine. Opiate alkaloids are known at times as narcotic analgesics because of the drowsiness and sleep (narcosis) which they can produce. (The term narcotic is now often misused to refer widely to any illegal drug or drugs of abuse in general, and it is therefore fast disappearing form the pharmacologist's vocabulary.)

Morphine and related compounds produce analgesia by acting on the CNS rather than at sites of tissue damage or inflammation in the periphery. They are able to produce an increase in patients' threshold to pain, and to increase their tolerance of pain. Opiate analgesics are powerful enough to suppress pain completely in most cases, but even when the pain is so severe that the patient is aware of it and is able to localize its site of origin, s/he is less concerned by it—there is a kind of mental dissociation between the presence and the experience of the pain. The centrally acting analgesics are able to control much more intense pain than the NSAIDs and are used primarily to relieve severe pain resulting from, for example, limb fractures, burns and tumours.

## Mechanism of action of opioids

### Opioid receptors

The ability of different opioids to produce a variety of different effects either on the CNS or on peripheral tissues such as the ileum and vasa deferentia led to the view that there are several distinct opioid receptors: $\mu$ (mu), $\kappa$ (kappa) and $\delta$ (delta). The $\mu$-receptors are activated by morphine and most of the potently analgesic derivatives such as fentanyl and pethidine (Table 9.1).

The $\mu$-receptors are responsible for the induction of analgesia at the level of the brain, but also mediate the respiratory depressant and euphoric actions of the opioids as well as the reduced gut motility and some of the sedation (Table 9.2). There is some evidence from the development of compounds such as naloxonazine, that there may be further subtypes of the $\mu$-receptor—a $\mu 1$ subtype responsible for most of the supraspinal analgesia and $\mu 2$ subtype mediating a degree of spinal analgesia, euphoria, constipation and respiratory depression.

**Table 9.2** Opioid receptors

| Receptor | Effects | Endogenous ligands | Transduction system |
|---|---|---|---|
| $\mu$ (mu) | Analgesia (supraspinal) ($\mu$1)<br>Respiratory depression ($\mu$2)<br>Euphoria ($\mu$2)<br>Sedation ($\mu$2)<br>Gastrointestinal inhibition ($\mu$2) | $\beta$-Endorphin ($\mu > \delta$) | 1. $G_i/G_o$ causing inhibition of adenylate cyclase<br>2. Increase of $gK^+$ |
| $\delta$ (delta) | Analgesia (spinal and supraspinal) | Enkephalins ($\delta > \mu > \kappa$) | 1. $G_i/G_o$ causing inhibition of adenylate cyclase<br>2. Increase of $gK^+$ |
| $\kappa$ (kappa) | Analgesia (spinal)<br>Dysphoria/psychotomimetic effects<br>Sedation<br>Inhibition of transmitter release | Dynorphins ($\kappa > \mu > \delta$) | $G_i/G_o$ closing calcium channels |

Naloxonazine is an antagonist at $\mu$1 but not $\mu$2 receptors. The $\delta$-receptors are also involved in many of these effects.

Kappa ($\kappa$) sites are activated by **butorphanol** and **pentazocine**, and seem to mediate some sedation as well as analgesia at the level of the spinal cord. The mechanism may include inhibition of the release of transmitters such as glutamate. Kappa agonists do not produce significant euphoria, and often produce dysphoria (unpleasant subjective feelings) which helps explain their low addiction potential (Table 9.2).

There may be at least two subtypes of the kappa receptor since some agonists open calcium channels while others, including dynorphin close potassium channels. Kappa ligands also show two distinct patterns of binding to neurons. Both subtypes can be blocked by norbinaltorphimine, which is a selective kappa antagonist. Another agent, U50488H, is a selective agonist for kappa-1 sites. A third site, kappa-3 has recently been identified in the brain, existing at a higher density than kappa-1 or -2. Its function is unknown.

The $\delta$-receptor can mediate analgesia at spinal cord level. These sites can be blocked selectively by naltrindole, and may consist of two subtypes, one of which the $\delta$2 is sensitive to a family of naturally occurring peptides, the deltorphins.

The sigma ($\sigma$)-receptor, to which pentazocine and butorphanol also bind, is now known not to be an opioid receptor at all. It was subsequently classified as a phencyclidine site—a component of the glutamate activated NMDA receptor (Chapter 4), but the term is now applied to a site of unknown function to which haloperidol can bind with high affinity (Chapter 6).

## Endogenous ligands

Electrical stimulation of the periaqueductal gray region (PAG) of the brain produces analgesia which can be prevented by the opiate antagonist naloxone. This finding, together with the discovery in 1973 of high-affinity binding sites for opiates in the PAG area raised the question of whether there are endogenous compounds related to morphine in the brain. A search for endogenous opioids was initiated in several laboratories around the world. In 1975 John Hughes and Hans Kosterlitz in Scotland isolated, from a large number of pig brains, fractions which had morphine-like effects on peripheral tissues. The active compounds were identified as two pentapeptides which were named **enkephalins**: leucine-enkephalin had the amino acid sequence Tyr-Gly-Gly-Phe-Leu and methionine-enkephalin was Tyr-Gly-Gly-Phe-Met.

It was soon pointed out that the sequence of met-enkephalin was embedded in the structure of a much larger protein released from the pituitary body and which was the origin of melanotrophic and corticotrophic peptides. This protein is known as pro-opio-melanocortin (POMC). It is now known that enkephalins are produced in several groups of neurons mainly from the precursor protein proenkephalin. Splitting of POMC results in the formation of intermediate-sized peptides such as $\beta$-endorphin (31 amino acids) which is the portion containing the metenkephalin sequence.

$\beta$-Endorphin is more potent even than morphine at the $\mu$-receptors and is considered to be their natural ligand. The enkephalins are in turn more potent than $\beta$-endorphin or morphine at $\delta$-receptors. More recently another group of opioid peptides, the dynorphins, have been identified. These are produced from the precursor protein prodynorphin, and are believed to be the brain's natural ligands for $\kappa$ receptors (Table 9.2). The different precursor molecules POMC, proenkephalin and prodynorphin are found in different sets of neurons in the CNS. $\beta$-Endorphin, for example, is produced at high concentration in the hypothalamus and periaqueductal grey matter of the hindbrain, while enkephalins are present in groups of small neurons in the dorsal horn of the spinal cord and in the striatum and limbic system. Dynorphins are found in the spinal cord and hippocampus.

The enkephalins and endorphins were shown to have analgesic activity when administered directly into the brain, and soon after the discovery of enkephalins many pharmaceutical companies embarked on programmes of research to produce non-peptide analogues which would be stable in the body and could be administered orally. It was hoped that analogues of enkephalins might lack the dependence potential of the foreign opiate alkaloids such as morphine. It has in practice proved difficult to produce suitable molecules, or to separate analgesia and dependence. It is possible, however, to inhibit the breakdown of enkephalins (though not selectively) by compounds such as **kelatorphan**, which inhibits peptidase enzymes such as enkephalinase. Such compounds are analgesic.

The endogenous peptides are almost certainly involved in pain control pathways in the CNS. Opioid antagonists such as naloxone can reduce the analgesic effects of placebo agents, stress and acupuncture, and these procedures raise the levels of opioid peptides in the cerebrospinal fluid. It seems likely that in all these cases analgesia is at least partly due to the release of opioid peptides which can then act on the relevant receptors in the CNS.

## Opioid drugs

Morphine itself (Figure 9.2) is still widely used for analgesia, although it also produces in many people a pleasant feeling of detached well-being, or euphoria. This is the basis of morphine's potential for addiction and abuse. **Levorphanol** is a close chemical analogue of morphine but tends to produce less sedation.

**Heroin** is the diacetyl ester of morphine and, although it is metabolized to morphine in the body, it has greater lipid solubility which allows it to enter the brain more rapidly and produce a greater 'high'. It is substantially more addictive than morphine with no pharmacological advantages. Its therapeutic use is restricted to the terminally ill, in whom some euphoria may help to ease their suffering and for whom addiction is a minor concern.

Besides analgesia, morphine depresses the sensitivity of the respiratory centre to carbon dioxide, an action which leads to respiratory depression. It also produces a marked general depression of the CNS (narcosis) seen usually as sedation and sleep at therapeutic doses, and reflected in the miosis (pin-point pupils) which results from the loss of cerebral inhibition of the oculomotor nerve. The combination of miosis and respiratory depression are strongly suggestive of opiate overdosing.

Opiates also suppress the cough reflex and thus find a use as centrally acting antitussive drugs. Morphine itself is not used because of its addictive potential, but its dimethylated derivative **codeine** (Figure 9.2), which has the same antitussive potency but causes less analgesia and euphoria, is present in many over-the-counter cough (and headache) remedies.

Morphine and its analogues exhibit a number of unwanted actions including the release of histamine from mast cells (causing itching, general vasodilatation and bronchial constriction). They also have marked effects on the gastrointestinal tract, inducing an increase of smooth muscle tone, but reducing peristalsis and thus causing constipation as a result of an inhibition of acetylcholine release from neurons in the gut wall. Although a nuisance when used as a analgesic this action is the rationale for the use of low doses of morphine to reduce diarrhoea.

## Opioid antagonists

Several derivatives of morphine act as antagonists of the opioids. **Naloxone** and nalorphine can both be used to reverse the respiratory depression produced by opioid analgesics, although naloxone is often to be preferred since it is a pure antagonist. Nalorphine is a partial agonist and, if respiratory depression is due to non-opioids or, for example, to the potentiating action of other agents such as ethanol, then its agonist activity may exacerbate the problem by increasing the depression.

## Non-opiate opioids

In attempting to separate the analgesic, euphoric and respiratory depressant actions of opiates, many chemical structures superficially unrelated to morphine have been synthesized. Phenylpiperidines include **pethidine** (meperidine) which resembles morphine in most respects except that is has much less effect on the gastrointestinal system. It does, however, have muscarinic blocking properties leading to the usual dry mouth and blurred vision. **Fentanyl** is around 100 times more potent than morphine in producing analgesia. It is rapidly acting and is used primarily as premedication for anesthesia.

**Methadone** (Figure 9.2) has properties similar to morphine, but with a much longer half-life of around 25 hours owing to protein binding. This slow rate of elimination has led to the use of methadone as a substitute for opiates during withdrawal from addiction. The slow decay of tissue concentration allows cells to compensate and withdrawal symptoms are consequently far less severe than with morphine or heroin withdrawal. Dextropropoxyphene is similar in chemistry and pharmacology but is less potent.

Of the benzomorphan series of morphine derivatives **pentazocine** (Figure 9.2) is the most frequently used. It has much less abuse potential than morphine, probably because of its partial agonist properties at $\mu$-receptors. It is also an agonist at the phencyclidine site on the NMDA receptor channel, which results in dysphoria and hallucinations, and at the haloperidol/sigma site. Pentazocine also has agonist activity at the kappa receptors which, as noted above, can induce marked analgesia with much less tolerance and dependence liability then $\mu$-receptors due to the production of unpleasant, dysphoric, feelings.

**Buprenorphine** is a thebaine derivative which is also a partial agonist at opiate receptors. The related compound, **etorphine** is around 100 times more potent than morphine but much longer-lasting. It has been used in the wild to tranquillize large animals for veterinary examination and marking.

## Structure–activity relationships

The structure of morphine, a phenanthrene based alkaloid, is illustrated in Figure 9.2. Simple modifications of the ring substituents have marked effects on pharmacological activity. Methylation of the ring A hydroxyl, for example, yields codeine, a drug with much weaker analgesic or respiratory depressant activity, or dependence liability, but good antitussive (cough suppressant) properties. The 3,6-diacetyl derivative of morphine is **heroin**, a drug with strong analgesic and addictive properties and fewer side effects (nausea and constipation) than the parent molecule.

Hydrogenation of the C7–C8 double bond in ring C reduces the analgesic potency of morphine and many of its derivatives (dihydromorphine, dihydrocodeine, etc.). The morphinan series of compounds lacks the ether link between C4 and C5 of morphine. **Levorphanol** is one such compound, whose properties are very similar to morphine.

Perhaps the most striking feature is that replacement of the N-methyl group of morphine by an alkyl group yields the partial agonist compound **nalorphine** (and converts levorphanol to the partial agonist levallorphan). The addition of a hydroxyl to C14 and a keto at C6 results in the full antagonist **naloxone**.

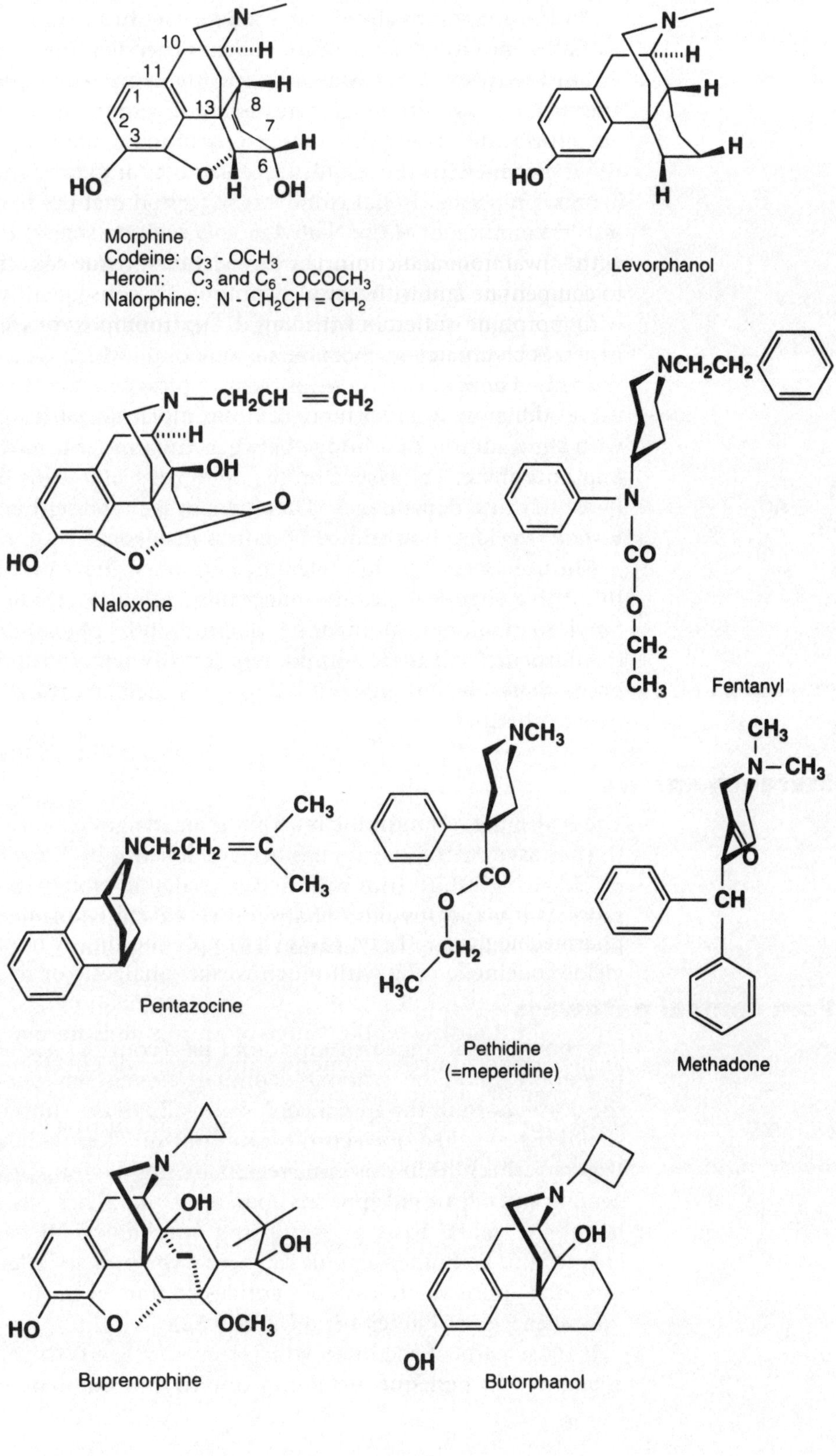

Morphine
Codeine: $C_3$ - $OCH_3$
Heroin: $C_3$ and $C_6$ - $OCOCH_3$
Nalorphine: N - $CH_2CH=CH_2$

Levorphanol

Naloxone

Fentanyl

Pentazocine

Pethidine (=meperidine)

Methadone

Buprenorphine

Butorphanol

**Fig. 9.2** Structural formulae of some centrally acting analgesic drugs.

An explanation has been proposed for the shift of properties from agonist to partial agonist to full antagonist. It is suggested that the opiate receptor exists in 'agonist sensitive' and 'antagonist sensitive' conformations, and that the presence of large N substituents increases affinity for the latter. In nalorphine, however, the N-allyl group can rotate freely in space, allowing some interaction of the molecule with the agonist receptor conformation and leading to partial agonist properties. In naloxone it is suggested that the hydroxyl group at C14 restricts movement of the N-allyl moiety such that the molecule is only able to act at the antagonist conformation, stabilizing it in this form and preventing attachment of agonist ligands.

Other modifications of the ring N substituent have yielded valuable analgesics. **Butorphanol** is a morphinan compound which is more potent than morphine and does not cause respiratory depression. It retains some tendency to cause addiction. A rather more complex molecule, derived from morphine but with the addition of a bridge between C6 and C14 making another ring, is **buprenorphine**. This is also more potent than morphine but seems much less liable to cause dependence. These two drugs represent encouraging progress towards the ideal non-addicting central analgesic.

The non-opiate opioid analgesics mentioned above may be considered to fall into three chemical classes—phenylpiperidines (pethidine meperidine) fentanyl, methadones (methadone, dextropropoxyphene) and benzomorphans (pentazocine). All these compounds actually represent fragment of the morphine molecule and Figure 9.2 illustrates their structures so as to emphasize their similarities.

## Stereochemistry

The (–)-isomer of morphine is active as an analgesic. The absolute geometry at the five asymmetric centres has been established by X-ray crystallography (5*R*, 6*S*, 9*R*, 13*S*, 14*R*) (Figure 9.2). Active analgesic molecules of other molecular series such as the benzomorphans possess exactly the same configuration at the positions equivalent to C13 and C14 of (–)-morphine.

## Pain control pathways

It is thought that some neurons form a pain control system in the CNS. Opioid receptors exist on the terminals of primary afferent neurons in external layers of the dorsal horn of the spinal cord, especially in the substantia gelatinosa, the site of the so-called nociceptive 'gate control' proposed by Melzack and Wall (Figure 9.3B). Within this same region are small interneurons which appear to contain and release enkephalins upon activation. These cells may therefore represent the neural basis of the 'gating' mechanism. It has been shown that enkephalins and other opioids can act on the primary afferent terminal receptors to suppress the release of peptides contained in those afferents, such as substance P (see Chapter 4 and Figure 9.3B).

If those parts of the brain which surround the IVth ventricle and cerebral aqueduct (the periaqueductal grey or PAG) are stimulated electrically in con-

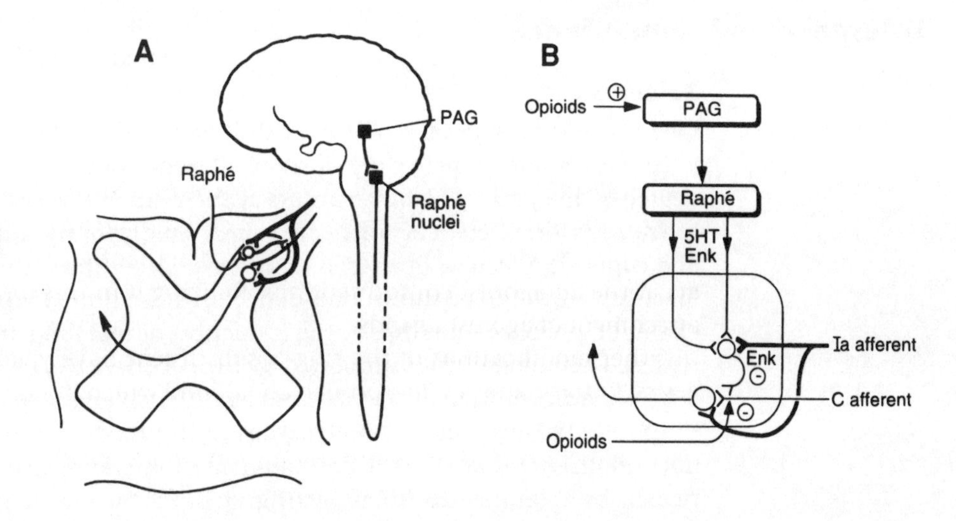


**Fig. 9.3** CNS pathways involved in pain control. (A) Neurons in the periaqueductal grey matter (PAG) project to the raphe nuclei, from where 5HT and enkephalin-containing neurons project to the dorsal horn of the spinal cord. There they synapse onto enkephalin-releasing interneurons which may suppress transmitter release from nociceptive C-fibre afferents, (B).

scious animals or humans, a powerful analgesia can be induced, in which there is a loss of noxious sensitivity from peripheral sites, with no loss of normal touch or temperature sensitivity. This analgesia can be reproduced by applying 5HT agonists into or around the spinal cord (intrathecal injection) and can be prevented by 5HT or opioid antagonists. It seems likely that an important pain control pathway therefore extends from the PAG to the raphe nuclei (Chapter 4) and that descending 5HT and/or enkephalin-releasing raphe-spinal neurons then descend into the spinal cord to activate the enkephalin containing interneurons (Figure 9.3).

In view of the wide distribution of endogenous opioid peptides in the CNS, it is probable that they are involved in more neuronal functions than pain control. The presence of a major striopallidal projection of enkephalin-containing neurons may explain the ability of natural and synthetic opioids to produce a depression of motor activity and catatonia (persistent immobility) in high doses. The presence of opioids in the hippocampus may explain opioid-induced amnesia, and their existence in limbic areas such as the nucleus accumbens may account for the euphoric effects of administration in humans. It has been proposed that it is a release of endogenous endorphins in exercise and stress which not only causes people to ignore major wounds (for example in athletes and soldiers) but also causes the feeling of euphoria and well-being which often follows exercise.

## Cellular effects

Although opioids are able to affect the activity of neurons in many parts of the CNS, few cell types have been studied in detail. In the locus coeruleus, for example, opioid peptides are able to inhibit cell firing by increasing potassium conductance. This will cause hyperpolarization and a secondary depression of calcium influx. It may be the latter effect which allows some opioids to inhibit the release of neurotransmitters such as acetylcholine from neuron terminals in the central and peripheral nervous systems.

# Tolerance and dependence

## Tolerance

One of the most serious problems with the opioid drugs is tolerance—the phenomenon whereby increasing doses need to be administered to maintain the degree of analgesia. Tolerance occurs at the cellular level and may arise at different rates for different actions: it develops rapidly for the analgesic, respiratory and euphoric effects of opiates, but hardly at all for the gastrointestinal effects. Since tolerance can be shown on isolated cells in culture it cannot be a pharmacokinetic phenomenon due to the induction of metabolizing enzymes in the tissues. This conclusion is supported by the occurrence of cross-tolerance, since different drugs tend to be metabolized by different enzymes.

Cross-tolerance occurs between drugs acting via the same receptors or transduction mechanisms (i.e. the development of tolerance to one agent is accompanied by tolerance to others acting at the same sites). Since all currently available opioid drugs produce analgesia primarily via the $\mu$-receptors, it is not practicable to restore efficacy by substituting one drug for another.

If cells in culture or isolated tissues are exposed for long periods to opioid agonists, there is evidence of receptor down-regulation, with a loss and internalization of receptors. However, changes of receptor binding sites have never been demonstrated in whole animals made tolerant to opioids. An alternative explanation is that receptors themselves remain unchanged, but they are uncoupled from second messenger systems such as G-proteins. This has been demonstrated in isolated cells and whole animals.

## Dependence

The term dependence refers to the compulsion to continue the administration of a drug without medical need. A distinction is often made between psychological dependence, referring to the perceived need some people feel for drugs reducing anxiety or producing sleep, or for drugs producing pleasant sensations or euphoria, and physical dependence in which withdrawal of the drug results in physical symptoms such as tremor, nausea and convulsions.

If morphine is withdrawn a rather unpleasant set of physical symptoms ensues, known as the withdrawal or abstinence syndrome. There are signs of autonomic overactivity such as sweating, lachrymation, rhinorrhoea, gooseflesh (hence the phrase 'going cold turkey' in addicts), increased blood pressure and heart rate, nausea and vomiting, severe cramps and diarrhoea. These are accompanied by marked restlessness, general irritability and aggression, tremors, muscle weakness and aching and insomnia. Throughout this withdrawal period (lasting around 10 days) the subject shows a strong craving for the causative drug, which may persist for weeks or months. Since opioid drugs can cross the placenta as well as into the brain, babies born to opioid addicts may show signs of withdrawal soon after birth.

The abstinence syndrome can be rapidly suppressed by administering the abused drug or a related compound acting at the same receptors. Conversely the syndrome can be abruptly precipitated by administering an opioid antagonist such as naloxone to tolerant individuals. One technique of minimizing the severity of withdrawal is to reduce dosage gradually and to substitute progressively with an opioid such as methadone which has a long half-life. The slow decline of plasma levels allows time for cells to adjust.

The administration of $\mu$-receptor agonists causes marked inhibition of cells in the locus coeruleus and withdrawal of opiates leads to a rebound hyperexcitability of these cells. It is not clear how important the locus normally is in the development of opiate dependence, but the administration of an agonist at the somatodendritic $\alpha$2-receptors, such as clonidine, which also depresses the activity of locus coeruleus neurons, can counteract the hyperexcitability of opiate withdrawal. Clonidine also suppresses many of the signs and symptoms of opiate withdrawal in humans.

The cellular basis of dependence is not understood with certainty but is probably related to the development of tolerance (Figure 9.4). A variant of the hypothesis presented above is that cells exhibit an overcompensation for the second messenger effects of opioids. One of the first examples of this was the finding that exposure to morphine inhibited adenylate cyclase, and thus reduced cellular cyclic AMP. Cellular adaptation by increasing cyclase activity soon overcame this effect of morphine, the dose of which needed to be progressively raised to achieve the same degree of inhibition (i.e. tolerance!). However, the cyclase still coupled to, and responded to, non-opioid receptors (e.g. for prostaglandins). When morphine was removed from the bathing medium, therefore, the cells were immediately hypersensitive to these other agents. This over-compensation mechanism may occur with other transduction processes too, and is very attractive because it may help explain drug dependence as well as tolerance; it is easy to understand on this model why reintro-

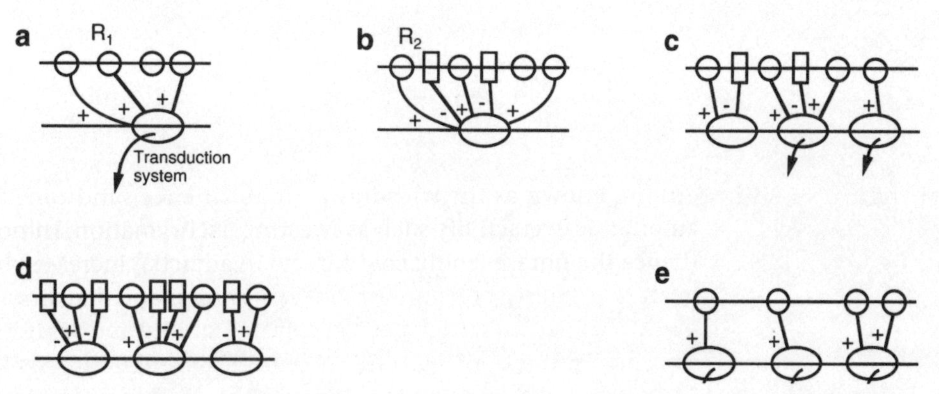


**Fig. 9.4** A possible mechanism of tolerance and dependence. In (a) an endogenous agent is considered to act at its receptors R1 (circles) to activate a signal transduction (second messenger) system. A drug may be used to activate its receptors, R2, (rectangles) and suppress activation of the system, (b). Some cells will respond to the presence of drug by increasing the amount of signal transduction components so that activity is restored (c). This necessitates increased amounts of drug to restrain the system (tolerance, d). If the drug is withdrawn suddenly the up-regulated signal transduction pathway is now free to respond to the endogenous agent, resulting in excessive second messenger and a withdrawal syndrome (e).

duction of the original drug will terminate withdrawal, since it will restore cyclase activity to its former state. An antagonist would displace the original drug and leave the increased cyclase available for stimulation by other endogenous agents thus precipitating a withdrawal response (Figure 9.4).

## Analgesia without dependence?

Although no drugs are presently available which have the ideal properties of inducing analgesia without dependence, it has been found that several groups of compounds can prevent or retard the development of tolerance or dependence to opiates without affecting analgesia. These agents include antagonists at the NMDA sensitive subtype of glutamate receptors, and inhibitors of nitric oxide synthesis. Also, antagonists at receptors for cholecystokinin receptors in the CNS will prevent the development of tolerance and yet potentiate opiate analgesia. Presumably, neurons releasing glutamate or CCK form part of the neuronal circuitry responsible for dependence. If it were possible to use combinations of opiates and any of these compounds, or ideally develop new molecules with hybrid structures active at opiate and glutamate or CCK receptors, then an ideal analgesic, non-addicting preparation may be obtainable.

# 10 Anaesthetics

## Introduction

The concept of general anaesthesia arose from the desire to mitigate the pain and suffering associated with surgery, and the fortuitous discovery around 1850 that certain agents (ether, chloroform) could produce a state of unconsciousness —a relative lack of reaction to stimuli and a concomitant period of amnesia. Before then patients were encouraged to take high doses of alcohol, cannabis or opium to subdue their awareness of the pain of surgery. The induction of unconsciousness also allowed surgeons to extend the duration and complexity of operations.

Modern practice has refined these two rather crude objectives, and aims to achieve control over a number of physiological variables—control of skeletal muscle contraction, prevention of autonomic responses to stress, maintenance of cardiovascular stability, suspension of cognitive functions, production of amnesia, removal of perioperative pain and anxiety etc. Anaesthetists use a cocktail of drugs to achieve these results; a mixture of around ten compounds is typical for a surgical operation. These may include substances capable of producing unconsciousness by themselves (volatile gaseous or intravenous anaesthetics), analgesics, sedatives, anxiolytics, muscle relaxants (neuromuscular blockers) and drugs affecting autonomic transmission.

Anaesthetics are classed as general or local depending on whether the loss of neuronal function achieved affects the whole body or merely a restricted region.

## General anaesthetics

Some authorities claim that several stages can be discerned during the induction of anaesthesia: (1) initial analgesia; (2) a brief period of excitement with signs of autonomic activity (coughing, salivation, hypertension) and muscle twitching; and (3) surgical anaesthesia. Phase (3) is rarely observed with modern anaesthetics. Deepening anaesthesia below phase (3) will lead to circulatory and respiratory collapse, and death.

### Inhalation anaesthetics

The compounds in this category are gases or volatile liquids which are administered by inhalation in air or oxygen at a sufficient gaseous partial pressure to achieve the necessary concentration in the brain. This critical partial pressure is usually stated in terms of the minimal partial pressure needed in the lungs to abolish sensitivity to a given noxious stimulus in 50% of subjects; this is the minimal alveolar concentration or MAC (effectively an $ED_{50}$ for anaesthesia). MAC is useful for comparing the potency of different anaesthetics.

MAC depends directly on the blood/gas and blood/brain solubility coefficients as well as the anaesthetic potency. The speed of induction of anaesthesia also depends on the solubility of anaesthetic in the blood, brain and other tissues. If an anaesthetic dissolves readily in blood its partial pressure in blood will be low and it will diffuse out of blood into the brain relatively slowly. If given at the same inspired partial pressure, therefore, anaesthesia will be induced more quickly by the hydrophobic drug, more slowly by the blood-soluble compound. This can be compensated to some extent by raising the initial inspired partial pressure of the blood-soluble anaesthetic.

As examples, nitrous oxide ($N_2O$) has a low solubility in blood (blood/gas coefficient = 0.5) and is thus able to induce anaesthesia rapidly, within 2–3 minutes. It also has a low lipid solubility. It therefore needs to be administered in theory at a high concentration (MAC 104%). Halothane on the other hand is about five times more soluble in blood, so that induction time is increased to 10 minutes or more. It is also about 150 times more lipid soluble than nitrous oxide and is therefore much more potent (MAC = 0.76%).

Note that anaesthetics are generally additive in their effects, so that half the nitrous oxide MAC (inspired partial pressure 52%) could be administered with half the MAC of halothane (0.38%), assuming no pharmocological or toxicological interactions.

Clearly the MAC will be influenced by many factors which alter the equilibrium relationship between alveolar and arterial partial pressures (bronchitis, emphysema, heart failure). MAC is increased for most anaesthetics by hyperthermia, alcohol and the presence of stimulant drugs; and decreased in the presence of other anaesthetics, and in hypothermia and pregnancy.

### Redistribution and duration of action

The brain, as well as organs such as the liver, kidney and heart, have a relatively high blood flow. Anaesthetics will, therefore, penetrate into these tissues relatively quickly. With maintained administration concentration will increase in poorly perfused tissues such as skeletal muscle and adipose tissue. Large amounts of lipid-soluble anaesthetic such as halothane can be taken up by adipose tissue, which will act as a reservoir of anaesthetic long after drug administration has ceased. Lipid-soluble anaesthetics therefore show a long duration of action.

### Effects of inhalation anaesthetics

With the exception of nitrous oxide, the inhalational anaesthetics are colourless, non-explosive, volatile liquid halogenated hydrocarbons (Figure 10.1). They all produce a variety of physiological effects other than, or associated with, anaesthesia including:

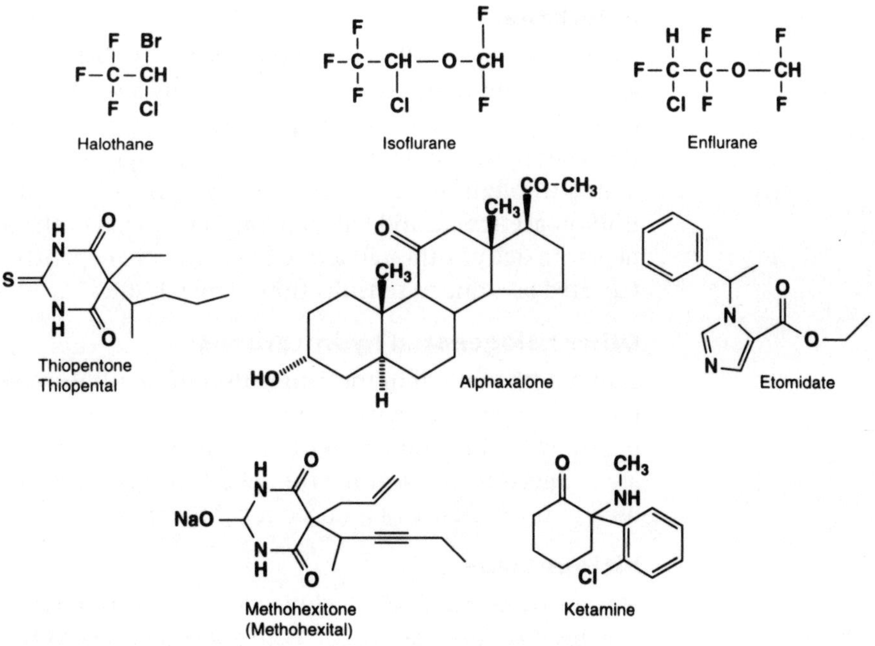

**Fig. 10.1** Structural formulae of some general anaesthetics.

(a) cerebral vasodilatation leading to increased cerebral blood flow;

(b) changes in the electroencephalogram (EEG). These are primarily related to the dimming of consciousness, but enflurane, at high concentrations can initate EEG activity resembling that seen in epileptic seizures;

(c) halothane can (very rarely) trigger cardiac arrhythmias particularly in the presence of catecholamine receptor agonists. These are usually benign and can be minimized by avoiding precipitating factors such as patient stress, inadequate anaesthesia, hypercarbia or exogenous catecholamines.

(d) halothane and enflurane (ethrane) have direct depressant effects on the heart, reducing contractility and cardiac output. Halothane also reduces coronary blood flow. The cardiac depression and loss of adrenergic vascular tone also results in systemic hypotension.

## The major inhalation anaesthetics

### Diethyl ether

Diethyl ether ($C_2H_5$-O-$C_2H_5$). This is now used mainly for short-duration surgery in small animals, since it is also a good analgesic and muscle relaxant. It irritates the epithelial lining of the respiratory tract, resulting in marked secretion of mucus which can lead to respiratory difficulties. It is highly flammable and explosive.

### Halothane

Halothane (Figure 10.1) is a potent (MAC = 0.76% v/v) and widely used general anaesthetic in humans, although it is only a weak analgesic at non-anaesthetic doses. It produces marked hypotension and cardiac depression, and sensitizes the heart to catecholamines, leading to arrhythmias. Halothane is mainly eliminated through the lungs, although around 15% is metabolized in the liver to trifluoroacetic acid and halogen ions. Even so, halothane does not seem to cause hepatotoxicity, although a rare idiosyncratic hepatitis has been described after repeated use, due to sensitization to metabolites.

### Other halogenated hydrocarbons

Like halothane, enflurane and isoflurane are halogenated hydrocarbons, and they resemble halothane in many respects. About 2% of enflurane is metabolized, with the production of fluoride ions and fluoridated metabolites which are believed to account for the renal toxicity occasionally produced. It is not used in the presence of reduced renal function.

### Nitrous oxide

Nitrous oxide has a relatively fast onset of action (low blood solubility) and is analgesic at sub-anaesthetic concentrations. Its MAC of 104% means that it must be combined with another agent to yield surgical anaesthesia (and leave room for some oxygen!). Its use is being seriously re-evaluated since the discovery that repeated use can disrupt methionine synthesis and thus disturb DNA and protein synthesis. This can cause blood disorders including anaemia on prolonged exposure.

## Injectable anaesthetics

In clinical practice it is very rare to use a single anaesthetic. Usually a balanced combination of agents is used to achieve: (1) a very rapid loss of consciousness; (2) a minimal amount of time in the excitement phase; (3) a stable plateau of surgical anaesthesia as rapidly as possible; and (4) appropriate levels of cardiovascular responsiveness and skeletal muscle relaxation for major surgery. While inhalational anaesthetics are useful for maintenance of stable, long-term anaesthesia, it is difficult to raise blood concentrations rapidly enough to fulfil (1) and (2). Anaesthesia is therefore induced using highly lipid-soluble anaesthetics which can be injected directly into the vascular compartment, and is then maintained by the inhalational anaesthetics.

### Barbiturates

**Thiopentone** (thiopental) and **methohexitone** (methohexital) are both barbiturates (Figure 10.1). The substitution of an oxygen atom by sulfur on the C2 carbon of the barbiturate ring renders the former highly lipid soluble. Both drugs induce unconsciousness within about 20 seconds of beginning an intravenous injection, mainly because of its very high lipid solubility which allows rapid penetration into the highly vascularized brain. Following the injection, however, blood and brain levels decline rapidly as the drug passes into tissues with a lower blood supply, mainly skeletal muscle, with which equilibrium is achieved in around 15 minutes. Despite the rapidity of induction, this redistribution of barbiturate would mean a rapid recovery from anaesthesia even though little has been eliminated or metabolized. Equally, the fact that skeletal muscle and adipose tissue will act as a reservoir of drug for tens of minutes (or even hours after a high dose) will result in a long hangover period in which the patient will remain drowsy and more susceptible to CNS depressant drugs. Since methohexitone is metabolized more rapidly in the liver, recovery will be more rapid. Like all barbiturates these intravenous compounds can produce marked respiratory depression.

### Etomidate

Although chemically unrelated to barbiturates etomidate resembles these agents pharmacologically. It is also metabolized rapidly in the liver, so that the dangers associated with a long hangover are lessened. It can cause adrenal suppression after repeated exposures.

### Propofol

Like etomidate, propofol is a rapidly acting agent used for anaesthetic induction and is metabolized in the liver. Patients are reported to recover from propofol more quickly than after any other anaesthetic.

### Ketamine

Ketamine resembles the hallucinogenic drug phencyclidine (PCP, 'angel dust'). Both produce a state of functional and electroencephalographic anaesthesia but with persistent eye and skeletal muscle movements. Patients may have their eyes open and be able to make some voluntary movement, but they appear unaware (dissociated from) their surroundings. This state is known as dissociative anaesthesia. It is accompanied by marked analgesia. Ketamine has some sympathomimetic properties and causes less cardiovascular depression than the barbiturates. Ketamine is among the safest of anaesthetics, causing little respiratory depression and leaving protective respiratory reflexes. It is a valuable anaesthetic when full hospital facilities are not available, as at the site of major natural disasters. It is also popular in veterinary medicine.

### Steroids

An additional group of compounds with general anaesthetic activity are steroids. Alphaxolone (Figure 10.1) and alphadolone are steroids, usually formulated for administration together (as Althesin) since this improves the solubility of the former, more potent compound. Anaesthesia is attained within about 1 minute of intravenous injection and lasts for 5–10 minutes. A useful degree of muscle relaxation is produced with some hypotension. Elimination is rapid, largely by liver metabolism, so that hangover is not a major problem. These agents are now mainly used in veterinary practice, having been withdrawn from human use following allergic reactions to the vehicle, but as the anaesthetic steroids themselves are relatively safe drugs, research is directed at producing similar compounds for human use. They appear to act by enhancing the inhibitory effects of GABA at interneurons in the brain.

## Mechanisms of general anaesthesia

There is a high correlation between the lipid solubility of anaesthetic agents and their clinical potency in producing anaesthesia (reflected in the MAC), suggesting that lipid solubility may be important for the production of anaesthesia (as well as the kinetics of induction and recovery). Meyer and Overton produced some of the early correlations between these parameters around 1900 (using cessation of swimming in tadpoles as a measure of anaesthesia!) and subsequently formulated a proposal that anaesthesia depended simply on the attainment of a critical concentration in cellular lipids. This hypothesis has been attractive for many years since it does not postulate a specific anaesthetic receptor which would be hard to reconcile with the simplicity and structural diversity of general anaesthetics.

One probable mechanism is that as anaesthetics dissolve in lipid membranes they cause a reversible expansion of the membrane which leads to a disruption of molecular interactions and thus depressed function. This idea is supported by the fact that pressure can reverse anaesthesia. If animals are anaesthetised and then placed in a high pressure chamber, the anaesthetic state disappears under pressures of the order of 100 atmospheres; the animals move about as if nothing had happened. As the pressure is reduced, anaesthesia returns until the anaesthetic is eliminated.

Attractive though this hypothesis is, it leads to a problem. If the anaesthetic potency of a series of compounds (such as some alcohols) is studied, it is found that increasing potency correlates well with increasing lipid solubility up to a point. Above a critical molecular size, anaesthetic potency declines very sharply even though lipid solubility continues to increase. This is very difficult to explain in terms of simple lipid solubility in membranes, as is recent evidence that anaesthetics interact with some form of saturable site in the brain.

A new hypothesis has therefore evolved that anaesthetics interact with a lipophilic (hydrophobic) site or sites on key cellular proteins, possibly ion channels or enzymes (Figure 10.2). The hydrophobic nature of the site would explain the Meyer–Overton correlations, while the critical effect of molecular weight can be explained if the site is of limited size. In fact there is some direct evidence to support this idea; at least one purified enzyme, luciferase (from fireflies) is inhibited by general anaesthetics with potencies correlating very highly with anaesthetic potency in mammals.

Other hypotheses for general anaesthetic action are now largely of historical interest. It is not likely that anaesthetics increase the fluidity of membranes (by diluting intermolecular interactions) since the same effects are produced by small increases of body temperature (which do not produce anaesthesia) and yet raising temperature actually reduces the potency of anaesthetics. Similarly the Pauling hypothesis that anaesthetics promote the formation of intramembrane hydrated complexes is unlikely; there is only a poor correlation between hydrate formation and anaesthetic potency.

### Site of action

It is likely that the effects of general anaesthetics are exerted mainly on the reticular activating system, the area of the medullary reticular formation mainly

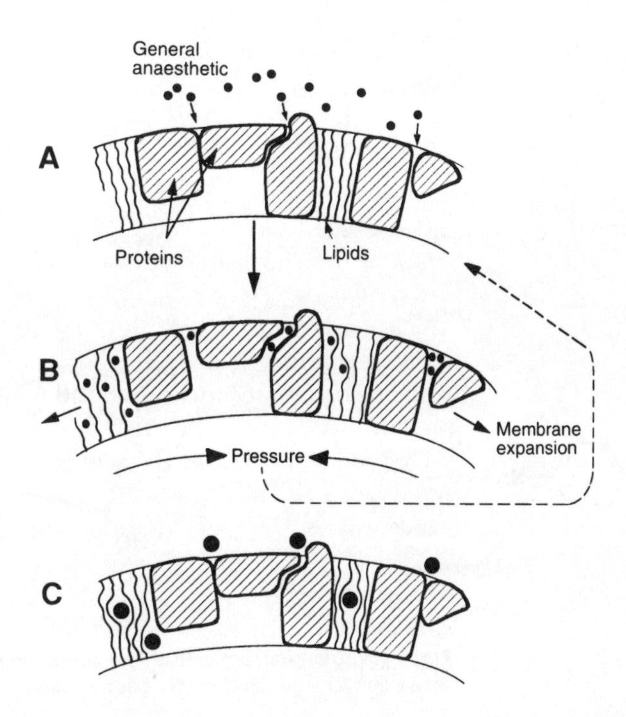


**Fig. 10.2** (A) A cell membrane consists of lipids and proteins. General anaesthetic molecules can diffuse into the membrane and interpolate themselves among membrane molecules to cause membrane expansion and a disruption of function (B). The application of pressure will eject the anaesthetic and restore membrane function. However, experiments show that above a critical size, molecules will still be able to dissolve in the membrane lipids but cannot produce anaesthesia (C). This suggests that it may be necessary for the anaesthetic to disrupt key parts of membrane proteins, which may be inaccessible to large molecules.

involved with the regulation of sleep and wakefulness. This is also an area rich in synapses and research has shown that anaesthetics depress synaptic transmission much more readily than, for example, axonal conduction. Excitatory synapses appear to be more susceptible to blockade, partly due to a reduction of transmitter release and partly due to a reduction of receptor channel sensitivity. Some of the injectable anaesthetics, especially barbiturates, markedly potentiate inhibitory neurotransmission by enhancing the ability of GABA to activate chloride ion channels.

Anaesthetics also have quite marked inhibitory effects on the hippocampus, especially by diminishing the release and sensitivity to acetylcholine. This may explain the amnesic effects of anaesthetics; most patients have difficulty recalling events associated with the induction and early recovery from anaesthesia.

The barbiturates are believed to act primarily by blocking excitatory neurotransmission mediated by the quisqualate AMPA receptors for glutamate (Chapter 4) and by enhancing the effects of the inhibitory transmitter GABA. Ketamine and phencyclidine (the dissociative anaesthetics) suppress excitatory neurotransmission by blocking the NMDA-sensitive population of glutamate receptors.

# Local anaesthetics

The first local or regional anaesthetic was cocaine (Figure 10.3). Chewing leaves of the plant *Erythroxylon coca* (for its stimulant properties) was known to cause numbness of the mouth. Cocaine was extracted from the plant as the active alkaloid in the late nineteenth century and was introduced for dental surgery

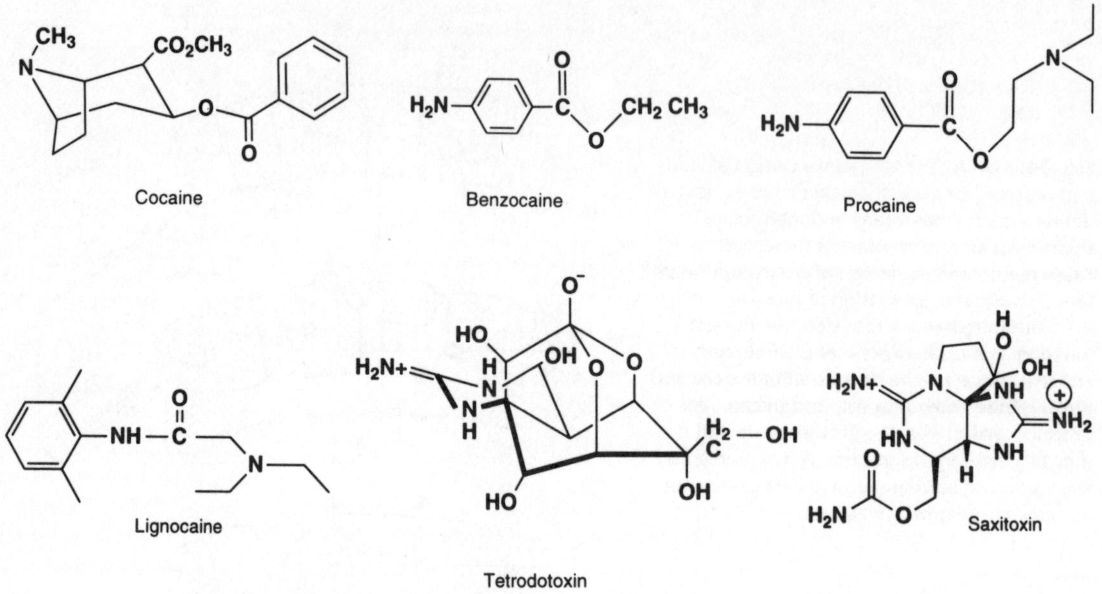

Cocaine

Benzocaine

Procaine

Lignocaine

Tetrodotoxin

Saxitoxin

**Fig. 10.3** Structural formulae of four compounds with local anaesthetic properties, together with the sodium channel blockers tetrodotoxin and saxitoxin.

around 1900. Since then a large number of chemical derivatives have been synthesized, most with the same basic structure of an aromatic nucleus coupled through either an ester or amide linkage to an amine side chain (Figure 10.3). They include benzocaine, novocaine, procaine and lignocaine.

In general the local anaesthetics block the conduction of action potentials in peripheral or central axons. To some extent this blockade can be reversed by high pressure, consistent with a degree of membrane disruption by expansion (see above) but the main mechanism of action is believed to be by blocking sodium channels. These channels can exist in an equilibrium between resting, open (activated) and closed (inactivated) states. Local anaesthetics bind most avidly to the inactive form, thus removing these from the equilibrium and shifting the equilibrium towards this form. The result is that most channels now exist in the inactivated form and axonal conduction is blocked. The blockade is greatly facilitated if neurons conduct a few action potentials soon after the local anaesthetic is applied, since sodium channels then cycle through the three states and become trapped in the inactivated form. This phenomenon is known as use-dependent blockade (Figure 10.4). Blockade of channels does occur more slowly even without action potential activity since the uncharged form of most local anaesthetics can enter the channels directly from within the cell membrane. This will clearly be the case especially for drugs with high lipid solubility. The blocking potency of drugs with poor lipid solubility will be much more dependent on use for them to gain access to the sodium channels via the openings.

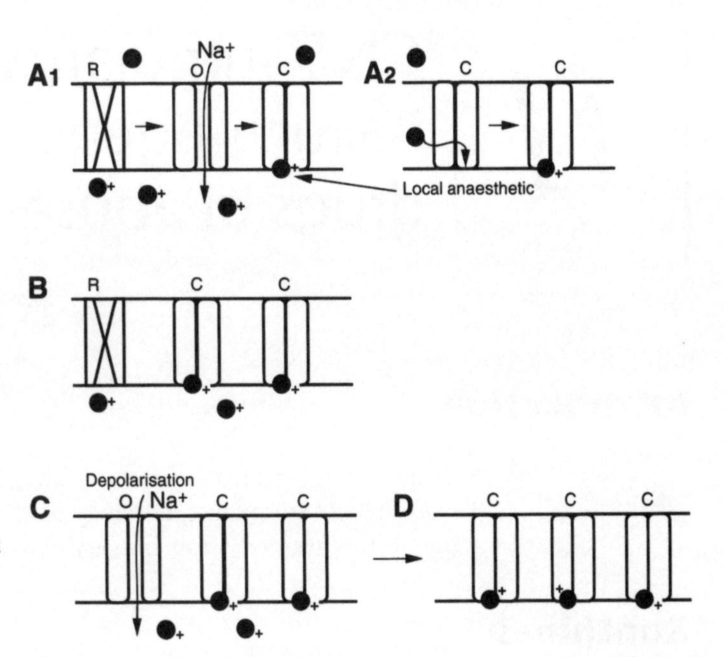


**Fig. 10.4** Mechanism of action of local anaesthetics. (A1) Sodium channels can exist and cycle between resting (R), open (D) or closed (C) forms, the open state being the conducting state during passage of an action potential. (A2) Local anaesthetic molecules can diffuse across neuronal membranes in their uncharged, lipophilic form, becoming ionized in the cytoplasm and blocking the internal portion of the sodium channel. Once combined with a local anesthetic, channels are held in their closed form (B). Since it is the open form of the channel which is most easily blocked, and the passage of action potentials involves the conversion of channels from resting to open states, the most active neurons will be inactivated more readily (C, D), a phenomenon known as 'use-dependent block'.

## Active Species

Most local anaesthetics are bases ($pK_a$ 8–10) and at physiological pH (7.4) they are largely ionized. However, they are inactive if applied to the outside of axons. It is the uncharged form of the molecule that diffuses into the cell cytoplasm where a new ionic equilibrium is established, most of the penetrating molecules then assuming the cationic form. It is this cationic form, acting on the inside of the axon membrane which blocks the sodium channels.

Local anaesthetics are used for the treatment of localized superficial irritations, either topically or by infiltration directly into the skin. They are also used for minor surgery or to block nerve trunks in the spinal cord (regional anaesthesia). They tend to block the small A$\delta$ and C sensory afferent axons associated with noxious stimuli more readily than the large A$\alpha$ fibres carrying fine touch and kinaesthetic information and mediating contraction of skeletal muscle.

## Tetrodotoxin

Although not used as a local anaesthetic, tetrodotoxin (TTX) (Figure 10.3) is frequently used in biological experiments to produce a blockade of sodium channels. It is produced by bacteria in the puffer fish, which is eaten as a delicacy in Japan. If not prepared correctly to remove the toxin this dish can cause death.

Another toxin, batrachotoxin from a South American frog, and the plant alkaloid **veratridine** have the opposite effect and promote the opening of sodium channels leading to persistent depolarization of neurons. After eating raw frog or *Veratrum* flowers, the end point is the same as with the puffer fish!

# 11 CNS stimulants, hallucinogens and other drugs of abuse

## Introduction

Drugs which produce an up-lifting of mood, or euphoria are sometimes referred to as psychic stimulants, and may be of value in helping to relieve mild depression during recovery from surgery or a bereavement, for example.

## Xanthines

Xanthines are derivatives of the purine nucleus and are met most regularly as the methylxanthines **caffeine** (Figure 11.1) and **theophylline** in coffee, tea and cola drinks. They are also included in some over-the-counter remedies for the symptomatic relief of the common cold and influenza, though the amount present (around 30 milligrams) is often equivalent to only half a cup of fresh coffee.

The stimulant effect of xanthines on the CNS results from their ability to block the generally inhibitory actions of the neuromodulator purine, adenosine (Chapter 4). This causes increased locomotor activity, increased alertness, insomnia and stimulation of medullary respiratory centre, an action which has led to the use of xanthines as respiratory stimulants in cases of infant apnoea. Effects on peripheral tissues result in tachycardia and diuresis. At very high, toxic concentrations some xanthines also inhibit cyclic AMP phosphodiesterase and trigger the release of calcium from intracellular stores. Together these may contribute to the hyperexcitability and seizures which are produced by toxic levels of the xanthines.

A number of other derivatives which are more potent and more selective antagonists at adenosine A1 or A2 receptors are being investigated for potential use in increasing attention, learning and memory in the elderly, confused or demented population. Drugs with these properties are known as cognition enhancing, or nootropic drugs.

## Drugs of abuse

Several groups of drugs such as barbiturates and some opiates that have already been mentioned in this volume, induce physical dependence after repeated use, and sudden withdrawal can lead to very unpleasant and sometimes life-threatening symptoms such as cramps, severe vomiting, seizures and coma. The definitions of drug abuse and drug misuse vary almost between individuals, but abuse usually refers to the habit of taking drugs in amounts or at a frequency beyond that necessary for a therapeutic effect. Drug misuse usually refers to drug use at a level at which the life style of the individual is disrupted and relationships with other persons are affected. Misuse may be considered equivalent to addiction, and may involve serious deviations in which much of the addict's time and energy is devoted to obtaining supplies of the drug in order to satisfy the craving and/or to prevent withdrawal signs. Note that a person may be addicted to a drug without necessarily showing marked signs of physical dependence. Conversely, a patient may become physically dependent on a drug such as an opiate after chronic clinical use, without showing any desire for the psychological effect of the substance.

Both addiction and physical dependence can be demonstrated in several animal species: rats and monkeys, for example, may perform repetitive tasks until totally fatigued, in order to obtain the administration of certain drugs.

## Nicotine

Nicotine (Figure 2.1) is absorbed from cigarette smoke or from the recently introduced gums and dermal patches containing the alkaloid. It is claimed by regular users to induce a stimulation of the CNS, but in new users, or in high doses, it can cause a depression of CNS functions. Even in low doses nicotine has a positive reinforcing effect in animals—they will produce appropriate responses, such as pressing a lever to obtain a shot of nicotine. The alkaloid presumably therefore produces subjective effects which are somehow pleasant, or rewarding, possibly helping to explain the addictive nature of tobacco smoking. Human smokers adjust the rate of smoking and the depth of inhalation in such a way that the plasma nicotine concentration is maintained quite constant, even if the nicotine content of the cigarettes is changed without their knowledge. Nicotine also triggers the release of dopamine and $\beta$-endorphin, both of which may contribute to the central stimulation and sense of well-being reported by habitual smokers.

Nicotine produces a variety of autonomic effects, including increases of heart rate and blood pressure, steroid release and catecholamine secretion. These are predictable consequences of stimulating nicotinic cholinoceptors at autonomic ganglia and adrenal chromaffin cells. It also reduces food intake, leading to a loss of body weight, probably as a result of its elevating blood glucose levels.

Tolerance rapidly develops to the effects of nicotine and chronic use can lead to dependence which is mainly psychological. The existence of some physical dependence is illustrated by the anxiety, depression, insomnia, restlessness, vertigo, tremor, irritability and nausea which may be experienced when the compound (or regular smoking) is stopped suddenly.

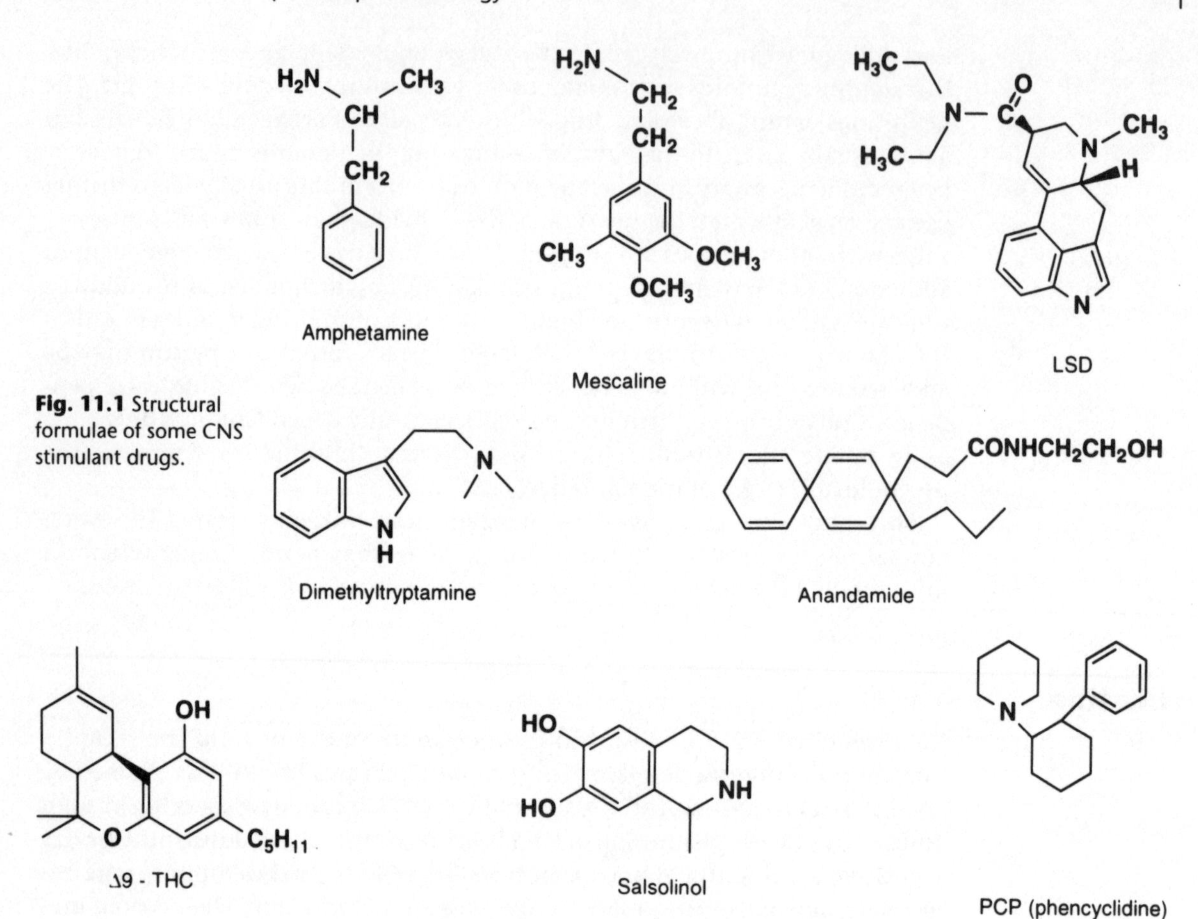


**Fig. 11.1** Structural formulae of some CNS stimulant drugs.

All the effects of nicotine can be prevented by drugs such as mecamylamine (Chapter 3), which can cross the blood–brain barrier and block nicotinic receptors in the CNS as well as in autonomic ganglia.

## Cocaine

Cocaine (Figure 10.3) is the active alkaloid in leaves of the coca plant (*Erythroxylon coca*) which have been chewed for centuries by South American natives to induce euphoria and relieve the tedium and fatigue of daily life. The intensity of the euphoria, the decreased sense of tiredness and the increased degree of alertness form the basis for its abuse potential. Common terms for cocaine include 'coke', 'snow' and 'crack'. The latter is one of the purest forms of cocaine available illegally. The rock-like lumps of crack may be heated until they melt and the cocaine vapour inhaled to produce rapid access to the CNS and an intense euphoria. The effects are relatively short-lasting, however, and addicts may need to administer a repeat dose after a few hours. Many animals will choose to self-administer cocaine if given the choice between it and food.

Even at low doses, cocaine can depress cardiac function, while in high doses it induces nausea and vomiting, increased blood pressure and cardiac arrhyth-

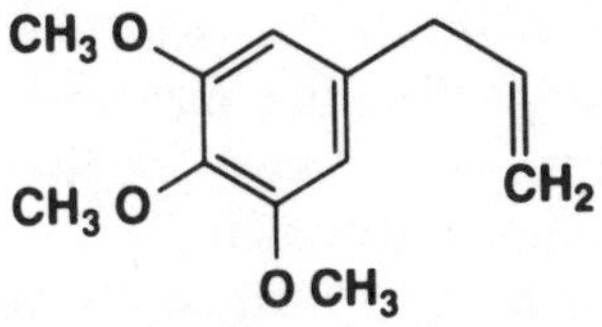

Elemicin

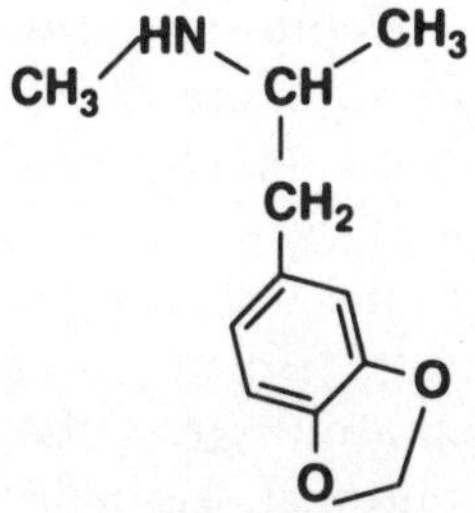

MDMA

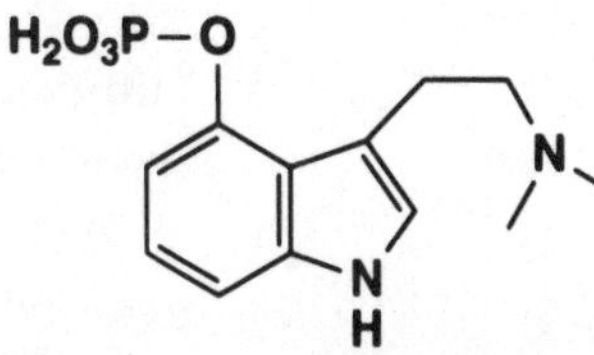

Psilocybin

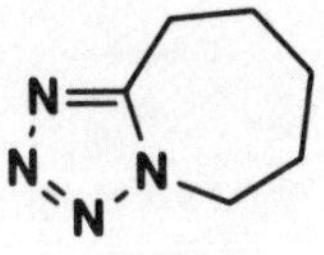

Leptazol

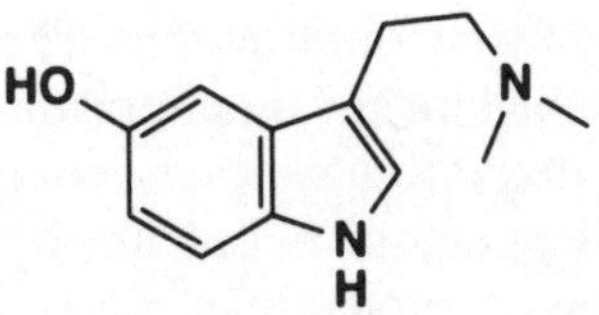

Bufotenin

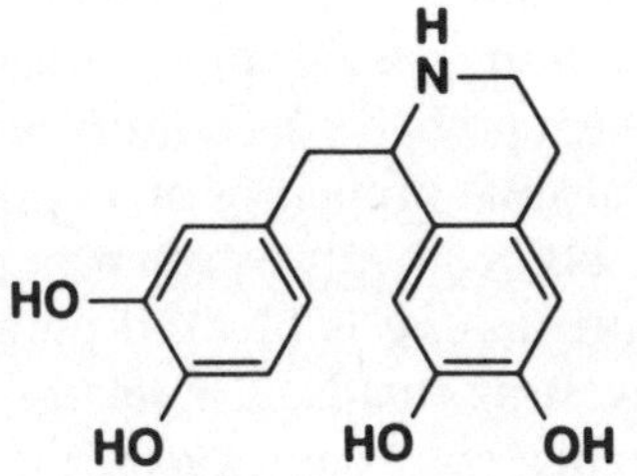

Complex isoquinoline

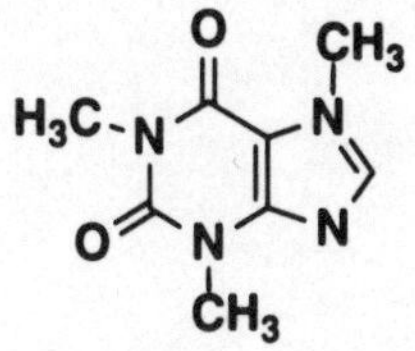

Caffeine

mias. It can also initially stimulate and then depress the medullary respiratory centre, and death not infrequently occurs from this cause, especially among intravenous users. Its euphoric effects are probably due to the inhibition of catecholamine uptake in the CNS. The marked addictive potential of cocaine may involve the activation of glutamate-releasing neurons, since NMDA antagonists can slow the development of dependence in animals studies.

Contrary to expectation, repeated use of cocaine seems to increase the sensitivity of most individuals, so that a given dose may eventually become a toxic dose, inducing a psychotic state with hallucinations and confused thinking similar to schizophrenia. Upon abrupt withdrawal of cocaine, subjects may experience excessive tiredness, insomnia, nightmares and depression. Although these symptoms can be extremely unpleasant and may persist for several days, they are not usually life-threatening.

## Phenylethylamines

This chemical group includes **amphetamine** (Figure 3.8), which is often abused because of its ability to raise alertness and attention, and to induce a mild euphoria. Together these factors can fool the unwary into believing, for example, that she is learning, or understanding, more than normal. Unfortunately this is not the case and many are the students who have entered an examination room only to find that they can remember almost nothing of a long night's work; the period following amphetamine use is characterized by a rebound loss of concentration and depression. Tolerance occurs with all the effects of amphetamines and chronic use can lead to a schizophrenia-like psychosis (Chapter 6). Psychological and physical dependence can occur, with withdrawal symptoms of increased sleep and eating, cramps, tremor and anxiety.

Although amphetamine and related compunds were used for their ability to suppress appetite in obese patients , their major clinical value now results from their paradoxical ability to decrease the activity of pathologically hyperactive children in whom the normal ease of distraction and lack of concentration represent serious limitations to learning at school.

Amphetamine is a typical indirectly acting sympathomimetic in the peripheral nervous system (Chapter 3) and it is likely that the various central actions of amphetamine are also due to the release of monoamines from nerve terminals. Catecholamine release appears to be mainly involved, with the neocortex and limbic system probably accounting for most of the behavioural actions. The euphoric and arousal properties of amphetamine can be blocked by pimozide, so they are likely to involve primarily a release of dopamine. The anorexic action of amphetamine is blocked by adrenoceptor antagonists but not by pimozide, suggesting that NA/NE release may be involved, probably in parts of the frontal cerebral cortex and amygdala.

### Dependence and self-stimulation behaviour

The topic of dependence to opioid drugs has been discussed in some detail (Chapter 9) but it should be commented here that dependence on amphetamines and cocaine is probably a direct result of their ability to potentiate effects of catecholamines in the CNS. If electrodes are implanted into the nuclei of origin of NA/NE or dopamine containing neurons, or in their ascending pathways (e.g. the medial forebrain bundle) then rodents will repeatedly press a bar to obtain electrical self-stimulation of those pathways. This will continue as long as stimulation is available, to the exclusion of feeding, drinking, and sexual activity, for example. Similar addiction can be produced by allowing animals to self-administer amphetamine or cocaine; dependence is not a uniquely human privilege!

## Analeptic drugs

A group of compounds known as analeptic agents produce a stimulation of the CNS without any euphoric or other psychological attendants. They are primarily antagonists of inhibitory amino acids and include strychnine (Figure 4.7) (a glycine antagonist), leptazol (metrazol, pentylenetetrazol) (Figure 11.1) and nikethamide. Even in quite low doses all these drugs may induce convulsions which can cause death due to muscle fatigue and respiratory failure. They used to find occasional use as stimulants of respiration (via the medullary centres) in cases of overdosing with depressant drugs but are now only of historical and experimental significance. Leptazol induced convulsions, for example, are a good model for the development of new drugs useful in absence epilepsy. Antiabsence drugs block these convulsions, though the relationship between them and absences in humans is not clear.

## Hallucinogenic drugs

Hallucinogenic drugs produce a distortion of the subject's sensory perception. The changes induced range (in most people) from mild changes of affect coupled with distortions of space and time (with cannabis), through to vivid, nightmarish and almost psychotic (psychotomimetic) episodes which may involve perceived threats, hopelessness, or commands to kill or commit suicide.

### Phenylethylamines

**Mescaline** is a phenylethylamine derivative (Figure 11.1) but, unlike amphetamine, it is believed to act directly on amine receptors, probably $5HT_2$ and NA/NE receptors, rather than by promoting release. It is present in the Mexican peyote cactus, preparations of which have been used since antiquity in religious and other rituals. Users may cut portions of the plant and dry them to form 'buttons' which are swallowed whole or powdered. Mescaline itself causes sympathetic stimulation (increases of heart rate, blood pressure, behavioural arousal, anxiety), unpleasant tremors, nausea and profuse sweating, and probably a metabolite is responsible for the hallucinations that appear several hours after administration of mescaline itself. The hallucinations often involve bright lights and geometric shapes, with distorted colour and space perception.

Related to mescaline are compounds such as **elemicin**, which is present in nutmeg and mace, common spices used in Western cuisine. Elemicin is rather weak, however, and large amounts would be needed for a 'trip' likely to be accompanied by severe tremors and vomiting. Cases of 'nutmeg psychosis' caused by ingesting huge quantities of the spice have been reported.

Another hallucinogenic amphetamine derivative, **methylenedioxymethamphetamine** (MDMA, 'ecstasy') (Figure 11.1) also affects 5HT neurons rather than catecholamines. After exposure to MDMA a few times , however, there is clear evidence for destruction of the 5HT-containing terminals in the cortex and elsewhere. It has been proposed that this may lead to serious mental abnormalities and psychosis in later life, but as MDMA is a relatively new drug, it will be some years before we know if this is true.

### Phencyclidine

Phencyclidine (PCP, 'angel dust') has been mentioned in other contexts (as a dissociative anaesthetic, Chapter 10), since it can interact with sites on the glutamate activated NMDA receptor (Chapter 4) and can interact with opioid compounds such as pentazocine at what was formerly regarded as an opioid receptor. It is not clear whether phencyclidine (Figure. 11.1) has other major sites of action, but when taken by humans in non-anaesthetic doses, it induces hallucinatory distortions of sensory perception, a profound sense of loneliness and can induce uncharacteristic episodes of violence in response to perceived threats. Coupled with pronounced analgesia some addicts may damage them selves. Different subjects experience euphoria or depression. PCP can cause seizures and cardiac arrest in moderate doses. Personality changes and sudden frightening flashbacks to previous life events can occur unheralded for months after a dose of PCP, and in some situations, such as when driving a vehicle, these may be hazardous.

### Indole alkaloids

After the preparation in 1943 of material from ergot (the fungus *Claviceps purpurea*) Hoffman reported strange sensory disturbances including objects changing shape, and visions with moving, brightly coloured objects. Some sounds were said to be 'transformed into optical illusions'. The cause of these effects was later identified as an indole alkaloid, lysergic acid diethylamide (LSD; Figure 11.1). LSD is active at an oral dose of 1 $\mu$g/kg, and is thus among the most potent agents known to affect the CNS. It readily crosses the blood–brain barrier and produces profound distortions of space and time, with vivid, often terrifying visual hallucinations. The crossover between the various special senses reported by Hoffman, in which different colours may trigger specific smells, or sound may have an apparent colour is a common feature of intoxication.

LSD is not especially toxic at the doses normally taken by users, though the hallucinations have caused people to commit murder or suicide, and to be involved in fatal accidents. The main danger of using LSD is the initiation of latent psychotic disorders, and flashbacks in which distortions of perception can occur quite suddenly, years after taking the drug. When the distortions occur at the wrong time, for example when driving a car, crossing the road or repairing a roof, the results can be disastrous.

Tolerance develops to these mental effects, but there is no evidence of physical dependence or abstinence signs on withdrawal. Many abusers do, however, develop strong psychological dependence, and repeated use can result in the development of serious psychotic disorders. There is some cross-tolerance to the effects of other psychedelic agents such as mescaline and psilocybin.

The similarity in structure between LSD (Figure 11.1) and 5HT (Figure 4.5) has intrigued many pharmacologists since Woolley and Shaw drew attention to it in 1954. In fact LSD can act at several 5HT receptors and produces, for example, a potent inhibition of firing of neurons in the raphe nucleus, presumably by stimulating 5HT somatodendritic autoreceptors. In fact the best correlation of oral *in vivo* hallucinogenic dosage and binding potency suggests strongly that the hallucinations are due to activation of $5HT_2$ receptors. Antagonists at $5HT_2$ sites might therefore be useful in bringing round an LSD-intoxicated individual who is proving violent or suicidal.

Drugs related to LSD include **dimethyltryptamine** and **psilocybin**, the latter being a constituent of several species of mushroom including **Psilocybe** which grows widely in central America. While about 200 times less potent than LSD, psilocybin is used by some central American groups in religious festivals. It induces similar spatiotemporal disortions to LSD.

Another indole alkaloid, **bufotenin**, is present both in certain mushrooms (e.g. *Amanita*) and the skins of toads (*Bufo* spp, hence the compound's name). It is also found in some South American plants, the seeds of which are ground and used as snuff. Besides producing marked visual hallucinations, bufotenin can induce very unpleasant motor effects including ataxia and paralysis.

## Cannabis

*Cannabis sativa* (hemp) is a plant and crude, crushed preparations of the dried flowers can be smoked or chewed in order to absorb a number of mind-altering compounds. The earliest references to the use of Cannabis are around 2700 B.C. and since then it has been used by most peoples of the world, in one form or another, and known as hashish, marijuana, bhang or ganja. Although mostly used by individuals, there are records which show that members of a bereaved person's family might throw dried Cannabis onto the funeral pyre, the resulting smoke being inhaled by all present and presumably dulling the sense of acute familial loss.

Prominent among the active constituents is **delta 9-tetrahydrocannabinol** ($\Delta^9$-THC) which is lipid soluble and easily enters the brain (or a foetus during pregnancy), producing a relaxed, disoriented state in which time seems to pass more slowly. There is a degree of euphoria too, (some people tend to laugh uncontrollably), sedation, decreased aggression and a loss of personal inhibitions. High doses can produce frank visual or auditory, hallucinations and during recovery from high dose euphoria, some subjects experience attacks of profound anxiety. High doses may also precipitate paranoid delusions, confusion and disorientation.

There is significant tolerance to the use of cannabis, although dependence is mainly psychological rather that physical. Nevertheless, repeated use of high doses results in clear withdrawal signs in some individuals, with restlessness, irritability, decreased appetite, weight loss and insomnia. At usual doses, however, Cannabis is relatively safe and most of the chronic respiratory problems associated with its use (bronchial irritation and inflammation, bronchoconstriction, emphysema) are mainly due to the inhalation of smoke particles. There is a continuing debate as the whether cannabis causes cancer, a possible consequence of its suppression of the immune system.

Although the precise mechanism by which the effects of cannabis are produced is unknown, a high affinity binding site for $\Delta^9$-THC, and its associated mRNA, have been identified in several regions of the CNS including neocortex and hippocampus. The binding site is coupled to adenylate cyclase and causes inhibition. This may represent the site of action of $\Delta^9$-THC and there is speculation that, as with the discovery of high affinity opiate receptors, there may prove to be a natural, endogenous molecule acting at the cannabinoid site. One potential such ligand has been identified as **anandamide**, (Figure 11.1), a simple amide derivative of arachidonic acid (arachidonylethanolamide).

Some constituents of cannabis extracts have therapeutic properties. Preparations of the plant have been used for centuries for their analgesic, antiemetic, anticonvulsant and antiasthmatic properties. $\Delta^9$-THC itself has marked anti-emetic and bronchodilatory properties and a synthetic derivative, nabilone, has proved to be one of the few agents capable of suppressing the vomiting which accompanies some forms of cancer chemotherapy. Some other cannabinoid analogues are analgesic. The objective in synthesizing new analogues is to try and enhance the desired therapeutic action while eliminating the potentially dependence-producing euphoria.

## Ethanol

Ethanol (ethyl alcohol, $C_2H_5OH$) has biphasic effects on the CNS of most people and animals. At low plasma concentrations, around 10 mmol/l, ethanol can produce behavioural or motor stimulation, reflected in decreased reaction time. However, there is an accompanying decline in performance accuracy and judgement; a subject asked to press quickly one of several coloured buttons to match a changing coloured light will respond more quickly, but will make more mistakes. Subjectively, however, s/he feels s/he has done better and that judgement is unimpaired by the alcohol; this is why driving after even small quantities of alcohol can be so dangerous. Ethanol also has an anxiolytic action at low concentrations.

The concentration window for these effects is small, and as concentrations rise, ethanol begins to depress cerebral functions. Attention becomes poorer, speech slurred and eventually incoherent, motor coordination is lost, learning and memory are impaired. These may be accompanied by a paradoxical elevation of mood and excitements as the balance between different neuronal systems is disturbed. At plasma levels around 100 mmol/l, most subjects fall into a coma, and death may occur due to depression of the respiratory centres in the medulla.

Ethanol has a variety of effects on systems other than the CNS, causing peripheral vasodilatation, increased steroid and gastric secretions and decreased secretion of antidiuretic hormone from the pituitary, leading to diuresis. Chronic alcohol intake can lead to liver damage and also to degeneration of the mamillary bodies projecting to the hippocampus. This condition, known as Wernick encephalopathy, is associated with a loss of short-term memory and with confusion (Korsakoff's psychosis) and is probably due to ethanol's retarding the absorption of vitamin $B_{12}$ in the intestine.

Interestingly, small to moderate quantities of ethanol (50 ml/day, equivalent to a pint of beer or half bottle of wine) can reduce platelet aggregation and decrease cholesterol deposition in blood vessels, possibly reducing the risk of heart disease.

The actions of ethanol on the CNS resemble to some extent those of general anaesthetics, and experiments on lipid membranes show the same kind of pressure reversal (Chapter 10). There is additional evidence for more specific molecular mechanisms. Ethanol can block the NMDA sensitive population of glutamate receptors, thus reducing neuronal excitability and, in the hippocampus, explaining the well-known amnesic effect of the drug (Chapter 4). Alcohol can also block voltage-dependent calcium fluxes through cell membranes, thus reducing the release of several CNS transmitters and depressing postsynaptic neuronal excitability. It can also enhance the action of GABA at its receptors, an effect which can be prevented by the benzodiazepine site antagonist flumazenil.

An action on the GABA receptor-channel complex may account for the cross-tolerance which occurs between ethanol, barbiturates and benzodiazepines. Lastly, ethanol inhibits uptake of the inhibitory neuromodulator adenosine; this may contribute in particular to the observed suppression of transmitter release.

### Tolerance and dependence

Tolerance to ethanol is partly metabolic, the liver enzyme alcohol dehydrogenase being induced with chronic alcohol ingestion, but is partly a behavioural adaptation. There is also evidence that the voltage-dependent calcium channels inhibited by ethanol up-regulate to restore pre-ethanol calcium fluxes. One result of this cellular tolerance is that cessation of ethanol intake by heavy chronic users leads to a massive calcium influx which may explain the occurrence of a withdrawal syndrome, with tremor, mental confusion, fever, nausea, hallucinations and seizures. This alcohol withdrawal syndrome is known as delirium tremens.

One neurochemical hypothesis for the dependence liability of ethanol is based on the fact that aldehydes can react chemically with amines. Acetaldehyde is a major metabolite of ethanol, and the condensation of this with catecholamines, for example, can lead to tetrahydroisoquinolines (TIQs) such as salsolinol (Figure 11.1), while aldehydes and tryptamine derivatives can yield $\beta$-carbolines (Figure 11.2). Both these groups of compounds have been shown to interfere with aminergic neurotransmission, and could play a role in the positive reinforcing properties of ethanol. It has even been proposed that, since acetaldehyde inhibits aldehyde dehydrogenase, more complex aldehydes might accumulate in the brain, such as the dopamine metabolite 3,4-dihydroxyphenylacetaldehyde. This can in turn react with dopamine itself to yield complex isoquinoline molecules related to morphine (Figure 11.1), some of which are claimed to increase ethanol intake after their administration to animals. None of these hypotheses are yet supported by wholly convincing evidence, but they do represent a tantalizing link with other drugs of abuse such as amphetamines and opiates.

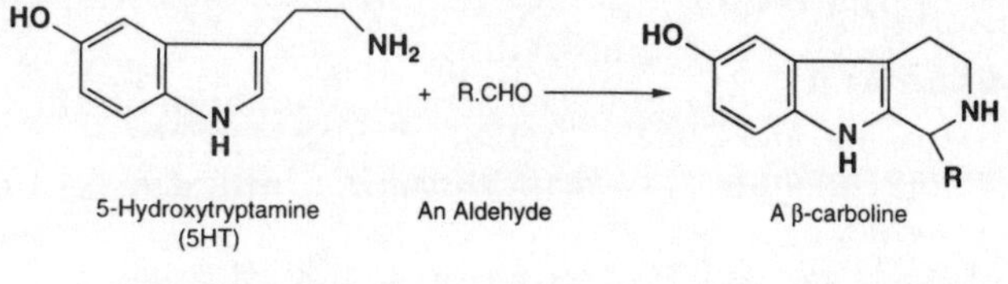

**Fig. 11.2** 5-hydroxytryptamine can react spontaneously with aldehydes in the brain to form $\beta$-carbolines some of which may have hallucinogenic properties (compare the structure of bufotenin in Figure 11.1).

# Further reading


**General texts:**

Bowman, W.C. and Rand, M.J. (1980) *Textbook of Pharmacology*. Oxford, Blackwell. Gilman, A. G. *et al.* (eds) (1990) *The Pharmacological Basis of Therapeutics*. London, Macmillan.

Rang, H.P. and Dale, M.M. (1993) *Pharmacology*. London, Churchill–Livingstone.

**Chapter 1**

Iversen, L.L. and Goodman, E.C. (1986) *Fast and Slow Chemical Signalling in the Nervous System*. Oxford University Press.

Lefkowitz, R.J. (1989) The new biology of drug receptors. *Biochemical Pharmacology*. **38**, 2941–2948.

Nicoll, R.A. (1988) The coupling of neurotransmitter receptors to ion channels in the brain. *Science* **241**, 545–551.

Stein, J.F. (1982) *An Introduction to Neurophysiology*. Oxford, Blackwell.

Various authors (1993) Molecular basis of ion channels and receptors involved in nerve excitation, synaptic transmission and muscle contraction. *Annals of the N.Y. Academy of Science*. Vol. 707.

**Chapter 2**

Bowman, W.C. and Rand, M.J. (1980) *Textbook of Pharmacology*. Chapter 17. Oxford, Blackwell.

**Chapter 3**

Gilman, A.G. *et al.* (eds) (1990) *The Pharmacological Basis of Therapeutics*. London, Macmillan. Chapters 4–10.

**Chapter 4**

Green, A.R. and Costain, L. (1986) *Pharmacology and Biochemistry of Psychiatric Disorders*. Chichester, Wiley.

Martinez-Rodriguez, M. (1994) Molecular and cellular aspect of neurotransmission and neuromodulation. *International Reviews of Cytology* **149**, 217–292.

Strange, P.G. (1992) *Brain Biochemistry and Brain Disorders*. Oxford University Press.

Webster, R.A. and Jordan, C.C. (eds) (1989) *Drugs, Neurotransmitters and Disease*. Oxford, Blackwell.

Various authors (1994) Receptor nomenclature. *Pharmacological Reviews* **46**, 111–229.

**Acetylcholine**

Caulfield , M.P. (1993) Muscarinic receptors—characterisation, coupling and function. *Pharmacology & Therapeutics* **58**, 319–379.

McGeer, P.L. (1984) Ageing, Alzheimer's disease and the cholinergic system. *Canadian Journal of Physiology & Pharmacology*, **62**, 741–754.

Stone, T.W. (ed.) (1994) *CNS Neurotransmitters and Neuromodulators. Vol. 1: Acetylcholine*. Boca Raton, CRC Press.

**Glutamate**

Stone, T.W. and Burton, N. (1988) NMDA receptors and ligands in the vertebrate CNS. *Progress in Neurobiology* **30**, 333–368.

Stone, T.W. (ed.) (1995) *CNS Neurotransmitters and Neuromodulators. Vol. 2: Glutamate*. Boca Raton, CRC Press.

**GABA**

Bowery, N.G. (1989) GABA-B receptors and their significance in mammalian pharmacology. *Trends in Pharmacological Sciences* **10**, 401–407.

Simmonds, M.A. (1983) Multiple GABA receptors and associated regulatory sites. *Trends in Neurosciences* **6**, 279–281.

**Purines**

Stone, T.W. (ed.) *Adenosine in the Nervous System*. London, Academic Press.

**Amines**

Bradley, P.B. *et al.* (1986) Proposals for the classification and nomenclature of functional receptors for 5HT. *Neuropharmacology* **25**, 563–576.

Carlsson, A. (1987) Perspectives on the discovery of monoaminergic neurotransmission. *Annual Reviews of Neuroscience* **10**, 19–40.

Various authors (1990) The neuropharmacology of Serotonin. *Annals of the N.Y. Academy of Sciences* Vol. 600.

**Peptides**

Hokfelt, T. (1980) Peptidergic neurones. *Nature* **284**, 515–521.

### Chapter 5

Ashton, H. (1993) *Brain Systems, Disorders and Psychotropic Drugs*. Oxford University Press.

Carlsson, A. (1987) Perspectives on the discovery of monoaminergic neurotransmission. *Annual Reviews of Neuroscience* **10**, 19–40.

Bradley, P.B. *et al.* (1986) Proposals for the classification and nomenclature of functional receptors for 5HT. *Neuropharmacology* **25**, 563–576.

### Chapter 6

Bradley, P.B. and Hirsch, S.R. (1986) *The psychopharmacology and Treatment of Schizophrenia*. Oxford University Press.

Carlsson, A. (1989) Current status of the dopamine hypothesis. *Neuropsychopharmacology* **1**, 179–203.

Ellenbroek, B.A. (1993) Treatment of schizophrenia: a clinical and preclinical evaluation of neuroleptic drugs. *Pharmacology & Therapeutics* **57**, 1–78.

Green, A.R. and Costain, L. (1986) *Pharmacology and Biochemistry of Psychiatric Disorders*. Chichester, Wiley.

Sokoloff, P. (1992) The third dopamine receptor as a novel target for antipsychotic drugs. *Biochemical Pharmacology* **43**, 659–666.

### Chapter 7

Bradley, P.B. *et al.* (1986) Proposals for the classification and nomenclature of functional receptors for 5HT. *Neuropharmacology* **25**, 563–576.

File, S.E. (1987) The search for novel anxiolytics. *Trends in Neurosciences* **10**, 461–463.

Sighert, N. (1989) Multiplicity of GABA-A–benzodiazepine receptors. *Trends in Pharmacological Sciences* **10**, 407–411.

Traber, J. (1987) 5HT-1A receptor related anxiolytics. *Trends in Pharmacological Sciences* **8**, 432–437.

Woods, J. H. *et al.* (1988) Uses and abuses of benzodiazepines. *Journal of the American Medical Association* **260**, 3476–3480.

### Chapter 8

Snyder, S.H. and Amato, D (1986) MPTP: a neurotoxin relevant to the pathophysiology of Parkinson's disease. *Neurology* **36**, 250–258.

Walker, M.C. and Sander, J.W. (1994) Developments in antiepileptic drug therapy. *Current Opinion in Neurobiology* **7**, 131–139.

### Chapter 9

Johnson, S.M. (1989) Opioid tolerance and dependence. *Pharmacological Reviews* **41**, 435–488.

Mansour, A. *et al.* (1988) Anatomy of CNS opioid receptors. *Trends in Neurosciences* **11**, 308–314.

### Chapter 10

Feldman, S.A. *et al.* (1987) *Drugs in Anaesthesia*. London, Arnold.

Rubi, E. *et al.* (eds) (1991) Molecular and cellular mechanisms of alcohol and anaesthetics. *Annals of the N.Y. Academy of Sciences* Vol. 625.

### Chapter 11

Kalivas, P.W. and Samson, H.H. (eds) (1992) The Neurobiology of Drug and Alcohol Addiction. *Annals of the N.Y. Academy of Sciences* Vol. 654.

Mechoulam, R. (ed.) (1986) *Cannabinoids as Therapeutic Agents*. Boca Raton, CRC Press.

Pratt, J. (ed.) (1991) *The Biological Bases of Drug Tolerance and Dependence*. London, Academic Press.

Smith, P.B. (1994) The pharmacological activity of anandamide, a putative endogenous cannabinoid. *Journal of Pharmacology & Experimental Therapeutics* **270**, 219–227.

# Index

## D



## E



## F



## G